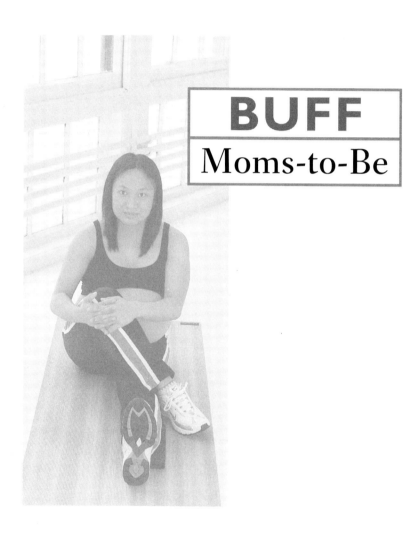

BUFF
Moms-to-Be

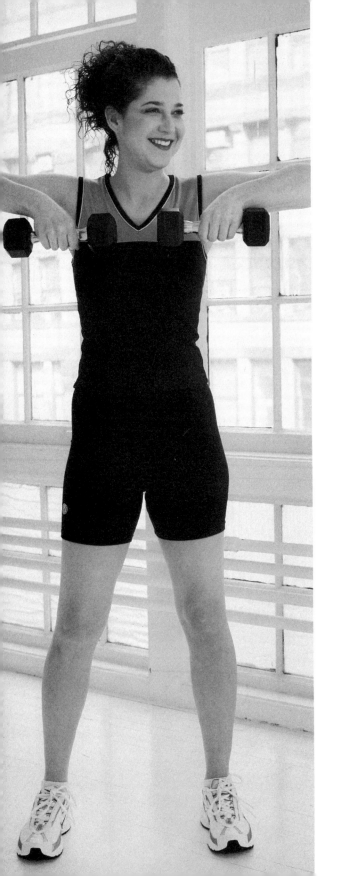

VILLARD NEW YORK

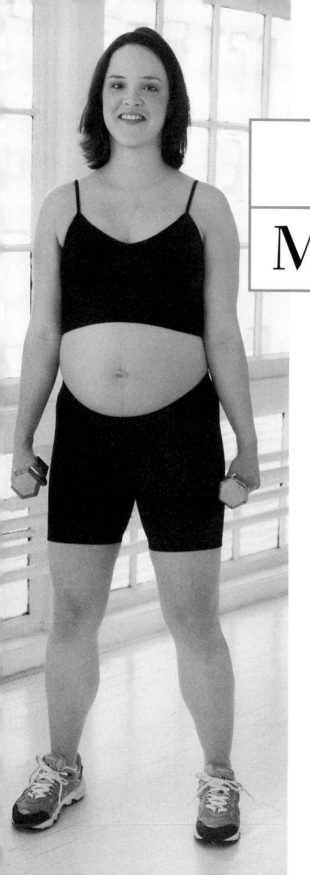

BUFF
Moms-to-Be

*The Complete Guide
to Fitness for
Expectant Mothers*

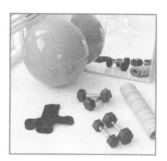

SUE FLEMING

Author's note: This book proposes a program of exercise recommendations for the
reader to follow. However, you should consult a qualified medical professional
(and, if you are pregnant, your ob/gyn) before starting this or any other fitness program.
As with any diet or exercise program, if you experience discomfort, stop immediately
and consult your physician.

Published in the United States by Villard Books, an imprint of The Random House
Publishing Group, a division of Random House, Inc., New York, and simultaneously
in Canada by Random House of Canada Limited, Toronto.

Villard and colophon are registered trademarks of Random House, Inc.

LIBRARY OF CONGRESS CATALOGING-IN-PUBLICATION DATA

Fleming, Sue
    Buff moms-to-be: the complete guide to fitness for expectant and new mothers /
    Sue Fleming
        p.   cm.
    Includes index.
    ISBN 978-0-8129-6945-0
    1. Exercise for pregnant women.   2. Prenatal care.   3. Physical fitness for
women.   4. Mothers—Health and hygiene.   I. Title.

RG558.7.F57 2003
618.2′4—dc21   2003050099

www.villard.com
Printed in the United States of America on acid-free paper
9   8   7   6   5   4   3

Book Design by Deborah Kerner/Dancing Bears Design

To the memory
of my father

Preface

LESLIE MILLER, M.D., AND

ALICIA SALZER, M.D. (IN PSYCHIATRY)

Congratulations! You have embarked on a miraculous journey. Pregnancy and motherhood are some of the most significant passages in a woman's life. As your body dramatically transforms to accomplish nothing short of a miracle, you may find that pregnancy and motherhood mark a period of spiritual awakening as well. It is a time when mothers begin to see their bodies in a whole new way. On occasion, you may feel like your body is on "autopilot," taking you on a journey with surprises around every curve. Sit back and enjoy the ride—your body knows what it's doing.

Now that you are pregnant, you undoubtedly are getting all kinds of unsolicited advice from everyone you know. But there is perhaps no aspect of a woman's life more riddled with superstition, old wives' tales, and plain old misinformation than pregnancy. The fact that you have bought this book means you are eager to enjoy the benefits that exercise in pregnancy affords but want a resource based on modern ideas and rooted in scientific research about what is best for you and your child.

There was a time when the pregnant woman was considered frail and fragile. In our mothers' generation, women were instructed not to raise their hands above their heads, lest the cord become wrapped around the baby's neck. Women often "took to bed" for rest and were protected from any physical exertion. As a vestige of these old beliefs, the medical term obstetricians still use to refer to your due date is your "D.O.C." or expected "date of confinement." Thankfully, pregnancy is no longer considered a condition requiring "confinement."

Being pregnant is often a powerful impetus for personal change. Knowing that your little one is growing inside you may be the motivating factor that inspires you to start an exercise regimen, even if fitness has not been a priority in the past. Based on an extensive review of scientific data, the American College of Obstetricians and Gynecologists (ACOG) published its most recent guidelines for exercise in pregnancy in January of 2002. The ACOG asserts that moderate exercise is beneficial in pregnancy for a variety of health-related reasons. This is true both for women who were previously active and fit as well as for women who have been sedentary or inactive prior to pregnancy. Before embarking on an exercise regimen, consulting with you physician is always the wisest thing to do.

According to the latest medical information that we have, exercise helps alleviate so many of the difficulties women experience while pregnant, from fatigue in the first trimester to back pain, constipation, and urinary continence issues later on. Some studies support the belief that women who exercise in pregnancy also deliver larger babies with higher APGAR scores (the APGAR score is a "wellness" score doctors assign to your baby in its first minutes of life). The idea that women who exercise deliver prematurely and have babies with lower birth weights and birth defects has been found to be untrue. On the contrary, moderate cardiovascular activity in pregnancy results in a decreased likelihood of delivering too early and has been shown to shorten the duration of labor and decrease labor complications. Exercise in pregnancy has even been found to play a preventative role in gestational diabetes and hypertension. Cardiovascular fitness during pregnancy is also linked to a quicker recovery after delivery.

In addition to its many physical and medical benefits, exercise also has tremendous emotional benefits. Cardiovascular exercise increases the body's natural "feel good" hormones—catecholamines and endorphins. Women who practice routine moderate exercise in pregnancy had lower scores on tests for depression and anxiety both before and after delivery. Research reveals that pregnant women who exercise regularly experience less social isolation and loneliness than those who do not. Most notably, exercise has been shown to improve women's self-reported body image, including muscle strength, body build, energy level, and self-esteem.

Yoga is great for meditation, while improving flexibility and relieving anxiety. It has also been shown that daydreaming about your unborn child and your future together helps you bond with your child, even before he or she is born. Pilates-type exercises are great for strengthening abdominal and back muscles that are essential to posture and delivery.

Pregnancy is associated with profound anatomic and physiological changes. There is much you will need to know about how your body is changing so that you can make smart decisions about how, when, and where to exercise. Your body mass, center of gravity, and blood volume shift drastically during pregnancy. Additional weight can stress the hips and knees, and the natural curve of your lower back, known as lordosis, may become accentuated. All of this becomes a source of both amusement and frustration as previously coordinated women find themselves becoming clumsy and even falling down more often. Exercise has been shown to improve a pregnant woman's coordination and balance. There is no better way to familiarize yourself with your ever changing body than to carefully and mindfully explore its new capabilities and limits.

Another muscular and skeletal change in pregnancy is your body's release of the hormones estrogen and relaxin when it starts to prepare the pelvis for delivery. These hormones loosen your ligaments (the things that attach your muscles to your bones), allowing the pelvis to widen, but also make other joints loose. So, although you may enjoy increased flexibility, you are also more likely to experience sprains and strains. Exercising helps to maintain the strength of your muscles so that injury is less likely to happen. When you exercise, you let estrogen and relaxin have their necessary effect on the pelvic ligaments, while preventing them from wreaking havoc on other muscles and joints.

When you are pregnant, your body consumes carbohydrates faster than it did prior to pregnancy, whether at rest or during exercise, so it is easy to become hypoglycemic. Building a baby calls for about three hundred extra calories per day after the thirteenth week of pregnancy, and that's not including any extra calories metabolized by your new or current exercise regimen. Low blood sugar for you means low blood sugar for the baby, and this is something to avoid. Never exercise to the point of fatigue or exhaustion. Those feelings may indicate that your blood glucose levels are getting low and will be too low for the baby. Make sure never to fast during pregnancy, and never exercise when you are hungry. It's also a good idea to wait an hour after eating before you exercise, so that your stomach, muscles, and baby won't be in competition for your blood supply and the carbohydrates and oxygen it's delivering.

The average weight gain during pregnancy is about twenty-five pounds. If you were trying to lose weight before you became pregnant, it's time to set those thoughts aside until after delivery, when you can approach weight loss with safety and renewed vigor. Pregnancy is never the time to lose weight, nor should you expect to maintain your weight or improve your level of fitness. There are studies that show that weight loss due to excessive exercise in pregnancy can cause your baby to be born with a lower than normal birth weight.

The weight gain and physical changes associated with pregnancy pose a particularly difficult challenge for women who suffer from eating disorders such as anorexia or bulimia. If you feel you may be suffering from an eating disorder, or have exhibited compulsive exercising in the past, it is wise to consult a doctor even *before* you conceive.

The same is true for women struggling with an addiction or substance-abuse problem, be it nicotine, alcohol, or recreational drugs. The first three months of a pregnancy are when the most important organs of the baby's body and nervous system are formed, and these kinds of addictions have been shown to cause birth defects. So don't think that just because it's early in the pregnancy, there's time to get those addictions under control later. Problems like eating disorders and addictions are often surrounded by shame and secrecy, and you may want to avoid discussing them with your doctor and loved ones. But it's important that you be frank with your doctor about your limitations. Minimizing the problem minimizes your doctor's opportunity to help—which *is,* after all, the reason we doctors chose to become doctors.

Since your metabolism is higher in pregnancy, your body-heat production is also higher. Expect to get hotter than usual when you exercise and also to perspire more. This is your body's way of trying to cool off. Anything that raises your body temperature more than a degree or two is off limits—that's the reason for all those NO PREGNANT WOMEN ALLOWED! signs you find posted near saunas and hot tubs. Be sure to wear loose clothing to allow your body to cool easily, do not exercise in hot, humid weather, and drink lots of fluids while you exercise.

Your body-fluid status during an exercise session can be checked by weighing yourself before and after the session. Any immediate weight loss is due to perspiration. Each pound you have lost during your workout represents one pint of fluid you need to drink to replace it.

Because of the increased metabolic rate and body heat production in pregnant women, exercise periods should be limited to fifteen to thirty minutes at a time. In the absence of either medical or obstetrical complications, it is suggested by the American College of Sports Medicine that pregnant women try to exercise on a daily basis, much like their nonpregnant counterparts. If you are new to exercise, start gradually and work up to thirty minutes a day. Even if you were quite fit before you were pregnant, you should not expect to continue the same fitness regimen you did before you were pregnant.

So now that we know how helpful moderate exercise can be in pregnancy, what exactly is meant by the term "moderate"? Moderate exercise does not stress or tax you. An easy rule of thumb is that you should always be able to speak comfortably while exercising. But the best measure is your heart rate. First start by calculating your maximum heart rate, or "MHR." The MHR represents the highest number of times your heart can beat per minute during periods of intense exercise. You can calculate yours by subtracting your age from 220.

Your target heart rate during pregnancy is a percentage of the MHR determined by your level of cardiovascular fitness prior to pregnancy. If you have *not* been exercising prior to pregnancy, you want to aim for a heart rate that is 60 to 70 percent of the MHR you just calculated for your age. If you *were* regularly exercising prior to pregnancy, you may aim for 70 to 80 percent of your MHR. So, if you are thirty years old, your MHR is $220 - 30 = 190$. If you want to work out to 60 percent of your MHR, simply multiply 190 by .60 and you will find that your target heart rate is 114 beats per minute. A little exercise goes a long way in pregnancy, so don't overdo it. Generally, a good rule of thumb is that if the mom is feeling it, so is the baby. Keep that in mind, and be aware of how your body is feeling during exercise. If you feel anything that is uncomfortable or stressful, stop exercising and consult your doctor before you begin again.

What types of exercise are best in pregnancy? Low impact, weight-bearing exercises are great for muscle strengthening. Swimming and walking are good ways to aerobically exercise. Activities with a high risk of falling, such as horseback riding or skiing, or those with the risk of abdominal trauma, such as football or ice hockey, should be avoided. Scuba diving and exertion at higher altitudes should also be avoided because of the risk of de-compression illnesses, which can cause major problems for mother and baby. As pregnancy progresses, changes in your body may limit what activities feel comfortable, and it is important to listen to those signs.

For example, a few months into your pregnancy you may notice it has be-come uncomfortable to lie on your back. There's a good reason for this. In this position your growing uterus rests on major blood vessels responsible for returning blood from your legs to your heart. If the weight of your baby presses on these vessels, the blood cannot return easily to your heart and therefore also can't continue on to your lungs, your brain, and your baby's pla-centa. As a result, your blood pressure drops and you may feel faint or dizzy. Therefore, after the first trimester, don't do exercises that require you to lie on your back. And after doing floor exercises, be sure to get up slowly to avoid dizziness.

Should you experience any of the following during exercise, stop and consult your physician:

Vaginal bleeding

Shortness of breath before or during exercise

Dizziness

A cold, clammy feeling

Headache

Chest pain

Calf pain or swelling

Abdominal pain, pelvic pain, or persistent contractions

Decreased fetal movement

Sudden gush of fluid from the vagina or a trickle of fluid
    that leaks steadily

Muscle weakness

Finally a word on the so-called baby blues. We all want to imagine ourselves as glowing and joyful moms and moms-to-be. But the reality is that 7 to 10 percent of women experience what they describe as radical mood swings during pregnancy. Irritability, elation, tearfulness, despair—all are frequently experienced for no discernable reason. Women who tend to have mood swings associated with their menstruation are more likely to have them in pregnancy. Avoiding caffeine, chocolate, and other concentrated sweets can help, as can talking with your partner or sharing the experience with other pregnant women.

In 10 to 16 percent of pregnant women, the severity of these swings begins to impair their ability to function and warrants professional treatment. Postpartum depression occurs in 10 to 20 percent of women and may have its onset anytime from giving birth up to several months after delivery. It is important to know that depression is treatable, and there are many forms of treatment that can be started while you are still pregnant. While most herbal or over-the-counter treatments for depression have been found to be unsafe in pregnancy, there are some prescription medications that are safe and can even be taken by breast-feeding moms. Other nonmedical approaches, such as light therapy, have been shown to increase the mood hormone serotonin and may help improve mood without medications.

Should you suffer from depression or other psychiatric illnesses before or during pregnancy, we advise that you consult your physician. The hormonal changes in pregnancy are known to exacerbate all psychiatric illnesses. Exercise is not a cure for psychiatric illnesses, and it has been shown only to be helpful as an adjunctive therapy for depression. Psychiatric illness such as bipolar disorder/manic-depression, schizophrenia, and schizoaffective disorder will require close psychiatric care during pregnancy.

While moderate exercise in pregnancy clearly provides significant benefits for most women, there are some women who should *not* exercise in pregnancy. This includes women suffering from medical conditions in which the baby's blood flow or oxygen flow would be compromised by exercise. Women with certain gynecologic conditions, which make the baby at risk for miscarriage, are also included in this group.

More specifically, women diagnosed with the following are advised not to exercise during their pregnancy:

Heart disease

Significant lung disease such as emphysema or moderate to severe asthma

Weak cervix (even if treated with the ringlike device called a "cerclage")

Multiple gestation (twins or more) at risk for premature labor

Low-lying placenta after twenty-six weeks gestation

Bleeding in the second or third trimester (threatened miscarriage)

Episode of premature labor during the current pregnancy, even if it has subsided

Ruptured membranes (your water has broken)

Diagnosis of pregnancy-induced hypertension

In addition, if you are diagnosed with one of the following medical problems you *may* be able to exercise in pregnancy, but *only* after getting clearance from your doctor and with ongoing medical supervision:

Severe anemia

Chronic bronchitis

Diabetes

Obesity

Extremely underweight (with body mass index <12)

Extremely sedentary lifestyle

Hypertension or preeclampsia

Seizure disorder

Thyroid disease

Heavy smoker

Intrauterine growth restriction in current pregnancy

If you are not suffering from one of the above conditions, it is likely that you will greatly benefit from remaining active and fit during your pregnancy.

Once your baby arrives, your life will undoubtedly be very busy. Research shows that women who don't begin an exercise regimen in pregnancy are unlikely to find the time to fit it in once the baby arrives. And it's not just a question of time; it's a question of a mysterious spiritual magnetism that makes us want to be there for the baby 24-7. Once again, evolution has left its mark, and we, as women, are neurologically hard-wired to feel we must prioritize Baby before all else.

Add to that our list of typical chores and responsibilities that range from work to caring for a partner to caring for other children and you've got one busy schedule. This is why many new moms refer to pregnancy as "the calm before the storm." So there is no better time to get in the habit of taking time to care for yourself than now, while you are still pregnant.

When you talk to friends who are seasoned at the art of motherhood, many may share with you that a common source of dissatisfaction with their lives is the perceived loss of self that comes with caring for others. The habit of making time for ourselves despite the cultural expectation of us as caretakers of others also requires practice. So start now.

Does all of this seem like a lot of information? Take heart. Since the dawn of mankind, the human female body has evolved to do just this. Whatever you are experiencing, from fatigue and nausea, to elation and a voracious appetite, rest assured that in the grand scheme, there is some adaptive reason for what you are experiencing that in some way benefits your baby. As you read on, you will learn more ways to optimize health and vigor for you and your baby. Have faith. Be well. Enjoy.

Foreword

SARAH HORTON KELLY, M.D.

My daughter was delighted when I told her that Sue Fleming had asked me to write a foreword for her book. Ann emphatically said, "She was the best coach I ever had." Ann, who played soccer, softball, and swam during her years at the Brearley School in Manhattan, knows coaches and knows that one who can inspire women to perform physically has a rare talent. Ann still goes for daily runs, is in great shape, and eats better than anyone else in our family. Sue and her program gave Ann the desire and the training to be healthy and fit for the rest of her life.

As I read over the manuscript, I got out my exercise mat and started stretching and bending. The book, the exercises, and feeling fit are fun. I am sure that you will find the book easy to follow and will be surprised at the breadth of the training. Sue outlines cardiopulmonary training, muscle strengthening, exercises for problem pain areas, and safe exercise programs. I know this book will encourage you to be active and fit during your pregnancy. Moreover, it will remain useful and beneficial for you for the rest of your life.

I have been in practice for more than twenty years as an obstetrician/gynecologist in New York City and have taught obstetrics for fifteen years. In residency I learned the term EDC, an acronym for the estimated date a baby would be born. The letter C stood for the word confinement, which pertained to the era when women were expected to stay at home during their pregnancy and after the baby was born. Now we know that exercise and activity are good for pregnant women. But traditional ideas and practices disappear slowly. Finally, in the last few years, the C is being replaced by a D for delivery, and women are beginning to know that exercise and physical fitness will not hurt their growing baby.

The American College of Obstetrics and Gynecology recommends at least thirty minutes a day of moderate exercise for pregnant women. The college simply warns against exercising to the point of exhaustion and against participating in activities that place the mother at increased risk of falling or of injuring her abdomen. They specifically discourage scuba diving because the baby can suffer from decompression sickness or the "bends" and warn against engaging in activities at altitudes greater than 6,000 feet because of the decreased oxygen content of the air. In other words, most exercise programs are safe to continue—or start. If you have any concerns about your exercise regimen, discuss them with your obstetrician.

The body goes through many changes during pregnancy. The cardiovascular system is dramatically affected. Blood volume increases by fifty percent to provide enough oxygen-carrying power for the mother and her baby. Muscle movement during exercise stimulates blood circulation, which is good for mother and baby. A pregnant woman who stands motionless for long periods of time is at risk of fainting because blood return to her heart decreases, causing decreased oxygen delivery to her brain. Working out reduces stress and anxiety and helps a mother manage the problems of pregnancy and her new baby.

There are many other advantages to your being a "Buff Mom": You will have more energy during your pregnancy. You will have a lower risk of getting gestational diabetes. You will sleep better at night. Labor will feel less exhausting to you, and you will be able to push more effectively when it is time for you to deliver your baby. Also, you will be able to bounce back from your baby's delivery faster and with more energy.

Sue gives excellent advice for how to deal with the emotional and bodily changes of pregnancy. She also gives good suggestions about diet and clothes. And the book has a terrific section on the postpartum period. It describes an excellent program for regaining your prepartum weight and form. Postpartum is a time when women often have the "blues." Exercise counteracts depression. Merely taking the time to do a workout will make you feel better about yourself. Furthermore, moderate weight reduction while nursing will not affect your baby's nutrition or growth.

Finally, being fit, healthy, and happy is the best gift you can give your new baby. Now go ahead—and start your training to be a "Buff Mom."

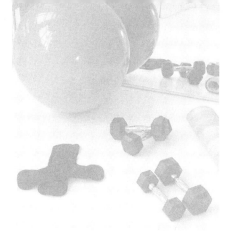

Contents

Introduction

The news is in, it's been confirmed . . . Congratulations, you are going to have a baby!

Motherhood is one of the hardest jobs on the planet. You will probably spend almost every second before you give birth thinking about the life growing inside you. You may spend the first couple of months full of excitement and absolute *fear* of having a baby—and you may tend to ignore some of the physical changes your body is going through. You may start to worry when it seems you can't control any of these maddening experiences: perhaps you woke one morning to find that your favorite pair of jeans doesn't fit. Food cravings become common. Your days revolve around when you will have your next meal. All of a sudden, the phrase "eating for two" hits home. Reality comes crashing in on you: "My body will not be the same."

"Will I be able to exercise safely during my pregnancy?" is a common question from many moms-to-be. Most of us grew up thinking that exercise was *not* safe for those life-changing nine months. Another common reaction is "Wait, I don't have time to fit an exercise program into my daily life." Suddenly, that maternal "glow" is gone.

When to start exercising *after* the baby is born is also a concern of every new mom. Postpartum exercise not only can restore muscular strength and firm up your body, it can also improve your emotional and mental well-being.

Doing the simple exercises I outline in this book can help tighten and tone muscles that have stretched during pregnancy.

That's why this book is for you. You can safely exercise during and after your pregnancy, in your own home, without investing a lot of time, money, or emotional worry. For many pregnant women, this is a time when they feel the most motivation to *start* an exercise program and feel good about it. And, finally, the word is out: doctors are on board with the fact that exercise is a *good* thing while you're pregnant.

My, how times have changed . . .

Here are some common comments heard in the doctor's office of the Stone Age:

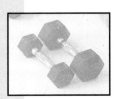

- "Don't move around too much." (OK, just sedate me for the next nine months.)
- "Don't raise your hands above your head and lift anything. You'll shift the baby and start contractions." (Does that include a blow-dryer?)
- "Don't lift anything heavy." (Does a pint of Ben & Jerry's count?)
- "Don't stand on your feet too long." (OK, I'll just stand on my hands instead.)

Scary but true: exercise was taboo for expecting mothers only until recently. Today, scientific research in favor of exercise has never been more convincing. A study published in 1995 in *Medicine and Science in Sports and Exercise* "found that women who continued exercising three times per week for thirty minutes or more at a moderate intensity gained *less* weight overall and put on less body fat than women who quit exercising during their pregnancies." Numerous studies have also found that women who exercised three times per week or more during pregnancy had shorter "pushing" stages of labor, less discomfort, less tension, and an improved self-image. Exercise may even lower the chances of needing a C-section.

Exercise can prevent potentially serious complications, such as high blood pressure. High blood pressure can lead to preeclampsia. Exercise during pregnancy may also prevent some of the aches and pains associated with carrying extra weight and changes in gait.

As a personal trainer who has worked with many mothers, expecting and postpartum, I constantly hear the concerns and questions of women trying to incorporate an exercise program into those ever-changing nine months. Perhaps you may never have exercised much before your pregnancy, or you were unable to follow a fitness program during your pregnancy because of health or other considerations. Whatever the situation, my book will help you during pregnancy, and help retrain your body after childbirth. I will focus on your most common areas of concern, specifically, flexibility; toning and strengthening the midsection; weight-training exercises to maintain strength in the upper and lower body; and lower-back exercises. This hands-on manual will challenge the myths of exercise during pregnancy. You *do* have time in your busy day to fit in effective, safe exercises that allow you to feel good about your body, release stress, and help you to feel and look healthier. Use this manual to have fun and enjoy the whole childbirth experience.

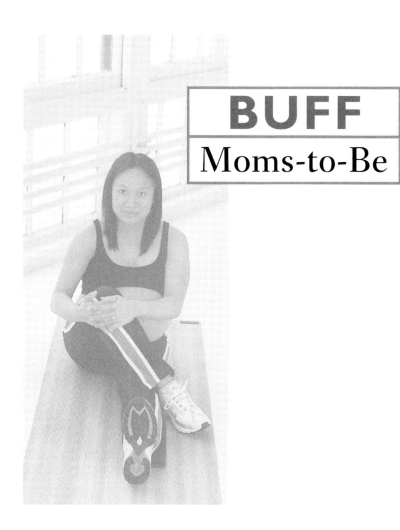

BUFF
Moms-to-Be

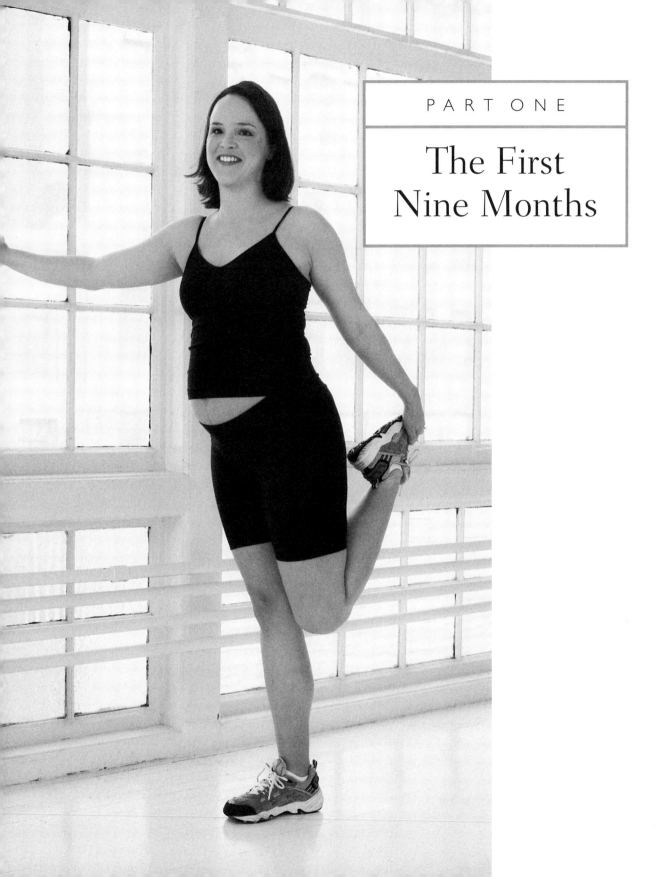

PART ONE

The First Nine Months

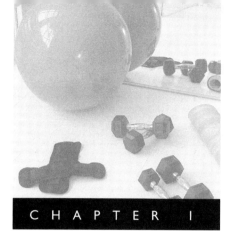

CHAPTER 1

Some Unique Considerations

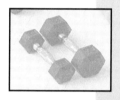

- The average woman will add 25 to 30 percent to her total weight over nine months.
- Pregnancy is an emotional roller coaster. Your hormones are raging.
- Stronger abdominal muscles are wider, longer muscles—*very beneficial during labor.*

BUFF BENEFITS OF EXERCISE DURING THOSE LONG NINE MONTHS

The Emotional Gain

When you're pregnant and bloated, why in the world would you want to put on an exercise outfit, look at yourself in the mirror, and work out? Believe it or not, exercise can actually help you feel better. Instead of thinking of the weight factor, think of exercise as giving you a needed emotional boost. Studies have shown that exercise releases serotonin, a chemical that can enhance your mood and lift your spirits. I've often heard that giving birth can be compared to preparing for and running a marathon. Preparing for your baby with an exercise program will make your birth that much easier, as you'll develop a sense of focus, strength, and determination.

Improved Energy Levels

Most likely your energy levels will be affected during pregnancy. Stronger heart and lungs, well-toned muscles, and increased flexibility will give you more zip during the day because you'll require less energy to do everyday tasks.

Self-Image

Many women are uneasy about the size of their bodies during pregnancy. Instead of focusing on this, get out and get active. Not only will it benefit your self-image, it will make it easier to lose the weight postpartum.

Sleep Better

It is quite common for women to have trouble sleeping during the later months of pregnancy. Exercising regularly is a great way to relax the body. But make sure you don't do a workout two to three hours before going to sleep, as the adrenaline from a workout can keep you up.

Improved Circulation

Circulation in the legs can be a problem for many expecting mothers. An exercise program can relieve varicose veins, swelling, and leg cramps.

Prevent Low-Back Pain

Strengthening the muscles of the lower back and abdominals can prevent some of the hip and back pain that women complain of during pregnancy. Low-back pain is common due to the extra weight you're carrying around.

AFTER THE BABY IS BORN

Transporting Your Newborn

A common complaint of new moms who didn't follow an exercise program during pregnancy is "I am so sore just carrying my baby around!" Remember, you'll also be carrying/pulling a stroller, a tote bag of goodies, and other baby accessories. Toning and strengthing the upper body (arms and shoulders) and the lower body (legs and back, for walking you and your baby up and down the stairs) is extremely important.

The Stretching Factor

So your belly has been stretched and pulled to a shape of unrecognizable proportions. Ah, to be able to fit into that bikini by summer. Well, as long as you give yourself ample time, that dream can be a reality. Daily exercise will help you attain your goal and help you feel good in the process.

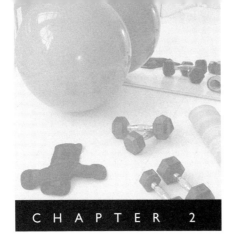

CHAPTER 2

Guidelines to Starting
an Exercise Program

Before you begin an exercise program, it is important to get approval from your doctor. According to the American College of Obstetrics and Gynecology (ACOG), there are certain conditions for which exercise is definitely not recommended:

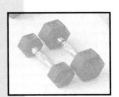

- Heart or lung condition
- Diabetes (There are certain conditions under which exercise is approved. Please ask your doctor.)
- Second- or third-trimester bleeding
- High blood pressure (pregnancy-induced)
- You have had three or more miscarriages.
- You are carrying twins, triplets, etc.
- Incompetent cervix (cervix is stitched closed)
- Rupture of the amniotic sac and leakage of fluid

For more helpful information, check out www.ACOG.com.

Once your doctor has given you the OK to exercise, be on the lookout for certain warning signs during your workouts. They are:

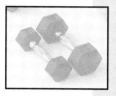

- Pain in the abdomen, chest, legs
- Nausea, dizziness
- Abnormal bleeding
- Heart palpitations
- Overheating, especially during the first six weeks

If you experience any of these signs, you should immediately stop your exercise program and contact your doctor or medical practitioner.

BODY CHANGES DURING PREGNANCY

Try not to beat yourself up if you find that you can't maintain the level of your old workout program. Modify your program and *listen* to your body. If something doesn't feel right, it's best to stop. Your body changes tremendously during these nine months, and that will alter your fitness regime. Let's look at some of these changes:

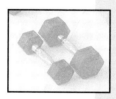

- Your uterus grows and grows to about a thousand times its normal size.
- Due to its increased size, your uterus pushes up on the diaphragm, and you may find a difference in your breathing. If you're used to going out for a four-to-five-mile jog, you may have to slow it down and shorten your distance.

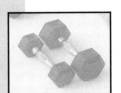

- Your heart enlarges. Your resting heart rate may increase by 15 to 20 percent.
- Obviously, your breasts enlarge. It's such an unfamiliar and uncomfortable feeling, and it can make a huge (excuse the pun) difference in your workout.
- Your stomach may go through some changes—a slowed digestive process can increase the chance of constipation. And let's not forget morning sickness. Nausea and vomiting are common because of all the hormonal changes.
- Since that enlarged uterus is now pushing on the bladder, your need to urinate may become more frequent. Sweating out excess water when you exercise can help reduce the amount of swelling one encounters during pregnancy.
- Due to the excess weight, your feet are killing you, and you find that they and your ankles are swollen!

And don't forget those hormonal changes . . .

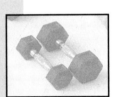

- You have an increased level of estrogen, which can cause water retention. Estrogen stimulates the growth of the uterus and breasts.
- You have an increased level of progesterone. This aids in the thickening of the uterine wall.
- You have an increase in the production of relaxin. Relaxin lubricates and softens the cartilage, ligaments, and cervix. This makes delivery easier. However, all this elasticity can affect

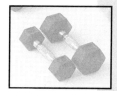

your joints, not just your cervix. Although you have more flexibility during this time, you are also more likely to have strains and sprains. Exercising will help maintain strength in your muscles so that you are at less risk for injury.

- You have an increased level of insulin. According to research, approximately one in three hundred women develop gestational diabetes mellitus. As stated earlier, if you have this condition, speak to your doctor about your exercise limitations.

- So great, your hormones are raging all over the place, your body is going through a major shift, what else can you expect? Ever hear about the PF muscles? Sure you have— the pelvic-floor muscles. Well, they too stretch and lengthen in order to allow the baby to come out. When these muscles are strong, delivery can be much easier. Strong PF muscles also help alleviate the common prenatal problem of urine leakage. That's because these muscles help control the bladder. Later in the book, we will talk a lot about specific exercises you can do to strengthen these muscles.

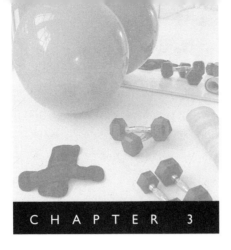

CHAPTER 3

What to Expect

THE FIRST TRIMESTER
(WEEKS 1 THROUGH 12)

The first trimester is an exciting time of your pregnancy. There are many changes that occur, for both you and your baby. If you have been working out moderately, continue with your program and add the exercises recommended in Chapter 5. If you've been sedentary, don't all of a sudden dive into a high-level exercise routine. Start slowly. Your body will be adapting to the changes of being pregnant. It is *not* recommended to have sore and achy muscles due to a strenuous exercise program. Try not to get overheated during the first six weeks, and try not to exercise on your back for extended periods of time. The ACOG advises women to stay off their back altogether during pregnancy. Supine hypotensive syndrome occurs when the enlarged uterus places pressure on the inferior vena cava (the vein that returns blood to the heart from the torso and legs), inducing nausea, dizziness, breathing difficulties, and a claustrophobic feeling. I tell my clients to listen to their body. If you feel OK on your back for short periods of time, that's fine. But once you feel the slightest bit of dizziness, roll over on your side and take the pressure off the vena cava.

Eating a balanced diet and staying well hydrated is crucial during pregnancy. Don't decide now is the time to go on a crash diet or one of those "diets of the week." During the first trimester, you will find yourself tiring easily. Let's face it, your hormones are going crazy with all of their changes, and that baby growing inside of you is very demanding. Its metabolic needs leave you exhausted. Motivating yourself to work out seems impossible. But once you get started, you will feel rejuvenated and happy that you mustered up the energy to exercise.

Another common symptom of the first trimester is morning sickness. Nausea commonly occurs in over half of all pregnancies. Hormonal changes, emotional factors, a slowed digestive system, and the growing uterus are all common causes. Morning sickness tends to worsen with an empty stomach and fatigue, so keep your eye on those two areas. Small meals and plenty of rest can help alleviate this problem. Ask your doctor about special prenatal vitamins if you experience morning sickness. Some women will experience more morning sickness than others. Try slow walks and lots of stretching. Take it one day at a time, and adapt your routine to how you feel. Some women find light exercise eases their morning sickness.

Listen to your body, and don't try to set personal records. Be flexible and adapt your program if need be. Again, avoid overheating and drink plenty of fluids (hydrating your body will help you regulate your body temperature). Keep away from high-intensity workouts. Most of all, try to enjoy yourself during your workouts. Remember, you're having a baby!

THE SECOND TRIMESTER (WEEKS 13 THROUGH 26)

Finally, you're starting to get used to the feeling of being pregnant. You feel better, you're more comfortable, and you may even feel the baby moving inside you. This is the time when you start to show, as well. Hopefully, morning sickness starts to fade, you have more energy, and you look forward to your workouts. Pay special attention to dizziness when you are lying on your back. Your uterus is thickening and growing now, putting even more pressure on the vena cava. If s/he hasn't already, your doctor may now recommend prenatal vitamins.

Since nausea has usually disappeared by the second trimester, you may have a renewed interest in working out. You aren't yet subject to the physical discomforts that may appear in the later weeks of pregnancy, and your energy level may increase because fetal organ development is mostly complete. By week 14, your baby is four and a half inches long and weighs about forty-five grams. Between weeks 18 to 22, he or she is quite active, and you will probably feel your baby move. Keep your workouts fairly intense and continue drinking plenty of water. Be especially careful during high-impact sports activities. Read Chapter 4 to learn which activities are recommended and which you should avoid. A diet that is high in fiber and includes plenty of fluids is encouraged now, as you may encounter some problems with constipation.

Some women may periodically feel their uterus tightening. These contractions, called Braxton Hicks, are harmless. You will probably continue to experience them throughout your pregnancy as your body prepares itself for birth. While Braxton Hicks are completely normal, if they occur more than four times an hour, call your doctor.

During the second trimester, your doctor should test you for gestational diabetes. A positive result should not discourage you from exercise; just make sure you discuss with your doctor any activities to avoid. If you have any of the below symptoms, be sure to discuss them with your doctor, as you may have a greater chance of developing gestational diabetes.

- Obesity
- Diabetes runs in the family
- Previous pregnancy with gestational diabetes

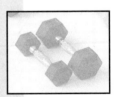

THE THIRD TRIMESTER
(WEEKS 27 THROUGH 40)

Hooray, the last trimester of your pregnancy! You're just getting the knack of having a super-duper belly. It's unusual to still have morning sickness, and I'm sure you don't miss that daily nightmare. Your baby is moving around more and more—sometimes it may feel like there is a kickboxing class in there! You find yourself making frequent trips to Baby Gap and putting finishing touches on the nursery. At about twenty-eight weeks, your baby measures around twenty inches and weighs about two-plus pounds. It is amazing how much growth occurs during the third trimester. Toward the end, the baby measures around twenty-six inches and weighs between six and eight pounds!

Since that belly of yours is quite big, it's no surprise that you are feeling a bit uncomfortable. Third-trimester moms-to-be experience insomnia—it's hard to find a comfortable position while sleeping. Exercise is an excellent way to find some relief. Now is the time you really have to listen to your body when working out. As long as you feel good, it's quite possible to exercise until the day of your labor.

Some of my clients report that they find it easier to breathe once the baby "drops"—no, not out of your body, but to the lower pelvis. This usually happens a month or two before delivery. Breathing is easier because there isn't as much pressure on the diaphragm as there used to be.

Relaxin, a pregnancy hormone, is responsible for the softening of the hip joints. As a result of the increased flexibility, you may catch yourself waddling. Also, the enlarged uterus throws your posture off, causing you to have a slight swayback. This can cause backaches throughout the final trimester. Strengthening and stretching the lower back will ease this discomfort.

All right, now that you know what to expect during those forty or so weeks, what kind of exercise program will make this time easier? What can you do to keep your body strong and prepared for the big event? The following chapters will outline, step by step, recommended aerobic, stretching, strengthening, and toning exercises you can do at home. These are safe, effective, and fun to do. Many women have found that doing these exercises made their deliveries easier and their postpartum recovery faster. Remember, everyone is different, so every body reacts differently to the dramatic changes you'll go through during the nine months of pregnancy. Doing these exercises will not guarantee you a simple, easy delivery, but the probability that it will help is great.

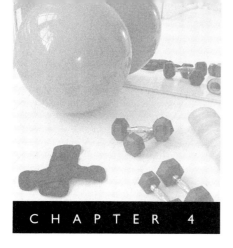

CHAPTER 4

Buff Mom
Guidelines

Befor you get started, carefully read the following exercise guidelines. I advise my clients to use common sense when exercising: don't try something that's unrealistic, and err on the side of caution.

- If you have *never* exercised before, get the OK from your doctor and start slowly. Keep a close eye on overexerting yourself and overheating.

- If you know the difference between a treadmill and a windmill, you should be able to maintain your exercise program throughout your pregnancy.

- So you're an exercise pro. That does not give you the OK to exercise to the point of exhaustion. When working out, make sure you can have a conversation and breathe easily. Remember, you have a baby growing inside, and he or she needs oxygen too.

Now's the time to treat yourself with some new exercise clothes. Wear comfortable, loose-fitting clothing. Stay away from the spandex. Invest in a good pair of sneakers that offer stability and support. And, please, don't forget the support bra.

Water, water, water! Before and after a workout.

Remember what I said about common sense? When choosing a sport or aerobic activity, don't do anything that can put you in a potentially dangerous situation. You may want to think twice about waterskiing and ice hockey.

Since your body is now releasing a good amount of relaxin, your joints may be a bit looser. Be careful of all activities that require quick changes of direction, stepping, jumping, and leaping. Any aerobic activities that involve rough, uneven surfaces should also be avoided.

Don't forget stretching. I devote a whole chapter to stretches that are beneficial before and after your labor.

The word "diet" should be removed from your vocabulary. Your menu should be chock-full of veggies, fruits, and complex carbohydrates.

Since you want to keep a careful eye on your heart rate, it may not be a bad idea to invest in a heart rate monitor. I have included the ACOG guidelines for the target heart rate for pregnant women in Chapter 5, as well as target-heart-rate guidelines for women postpartum.

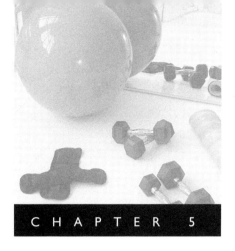

Getting Started:
Safe Aerobic Exercises to Enjoy
During Your Pregnancy

An effective workout is a balanced workout. Varying your cardiovascular routine will not only prevent boredom, it will allow your body to burn calories more efficiently and keep your heart and lungs strong. Stretching, cardiovascular activities, and strength training are the three elements of a fitness routine that will yield positive results. As you progress in your pregnancy, it will be hard to maintain your current cardiovascular routine. *That's OK!* Don't try to do what you were capable of before you were pregnant. On the other hand, some of my clients dislike incorporating any activity that gets them moving and shaking. Excuses such as "I don't have time" or "I don't like to run" are common. News flash: there are many safe, effective activities that strengthen the heart and lungs that are fun and easy to do. Don't set yourself up for failure. Find a couple of things you like to do, and you'll be more likely to stick with the program.

Before I outline safe and unsafe activities, I would like to talk about your target-heart-rate zone.

➤ If you choose to do strenuous exercise (only for those who are physically fit prior to pregnancy), it should be limited to fifteen minutes.

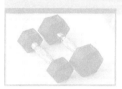

TARGET HEART RATE

When you're pregnant, it's especially important not to exceed the recommended target heart rate. Basically, reaching your target heart rate means exercising so that your heart beats at the level that gives you the best workout. When you exercise, not only does your external body temperature rise, so does your internal temperature. Your internal body temperature is a few degrees warmer than your external because there isn't an internal cooling mechanism. Your baby's temperature can rise to unsafe levels if you don't regulate your activities. Until recently, the ACOG recommended that you should not let your heart rate exceed 140 beats per minute while exercising. In 2002, the ACOG released new guidelines indicating that there is no proof that exceeding 140 is unsafe. Many experts are now adopting Borg's Scale of Perceived Exertion. Basically, this states that the intensity of your exercise program may be how hard you perceive your exertion to be. During pregnancy, your exercise intensity should be light to moderate, or in the range of 11 to 14, 6 being the lowest and 20 being the highest. Generally, for beginners, it is recommended to exercise at 60 percent of your maximum heart rate combined with a lower exertion level. Since your heart will increase in size as you progress in your pregnancy, relying on just your heart rate is not recommended. Again, if you feel weak and breathless during a workout, slow it down, and *never* work to the point of exhaustion.

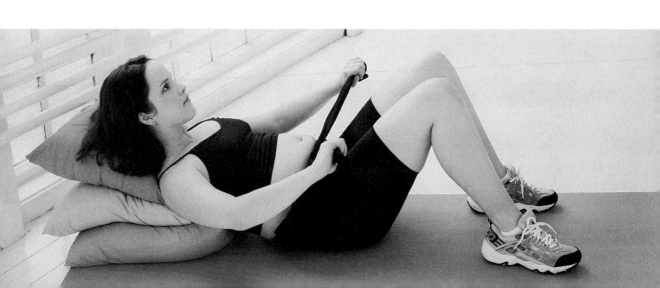

BORG PERCEIVED EXERTION SCALE

The Borg Perceived Exertion Scale gives you an idea of how hard exercising should feel. If it feels light (less than 12), you should increase the pace of your walking, biking, swimming, etc. If the exercise feels hard (14 or higher), you need to slow the pace. Exercise should feel somewhat hard (11 to 14 if you're pregnant).

BORG'S SCALE:

6	
7	very, very light
8	
9	very light
10	
11	fairly light
12	
13	somewhat hard
14	
15	hard
16	
17	very hard
18	
19	very, very hard
20	

It is also recommended that a cardiovascular workout not exceed forty minutes. This may be hard for the fitness fanatic. It's better to break up your workouts into two thirty-minute sessions (one morning, one later during the day) than to go for one hour straight. As I discussed in the previous chapter, wearing loose clothing with plenty of ventilation is extremely important in keeping the core body temperature in a safe zone. Of course, plenty of water will not only regulate your body temperature, it will also replace the fluids lost during exercise. It's not a bad idea to double your water intake as you continue to work out. I advise you not to work out during extremely hot weather. Avoid the dog days of August.

Most important, the nine months of pregnancy are not a time to achieve monumental fitness goals. Maintaining your fitness and staying healthy should be your priorities. Listen to your body and adapt your workouts to this sensitive time of your life.

Here is a simple formula for determining your target heart rate (THR):

You can easily take your pulse, or find your heart rate, at the wrist or heart. First you must find out what your maximum heart rate is (MHR), or the maximum number of times your heart beats in one minute.

To determine your MHR:

$$220 - age = MHR$$

You can then figure your THR by calculating 60 percent of your MHR.

For example, for a twenty-six-year-old woman:

$$MHR: 220 - 26 = 194$$

$$THR\ (60\%): 194 \times .60 = 115.4$$

As I stated earlier, if you are just starting an exercise program, take it slow. You may find it difficult to stay in your target-heart-rate zone. If you have more exercise experience, you may be able to work out a bit harder. Just keep your eye on the 140-beats-per-minute zone and your perceived level of exhaustion. Using a heart rate monitor ensures that you will not reach a dangerous level. You can also check your heart rate manually, although this is not as accurate. Periodically, during your workout, place your index and middle fingers in the groove on the side of your throat (don't use your thumb). Starting at zero, count how many times your heart beats in six seconds. Add a zero to that number. This is how many times (approximately) your heart is beating in one minute.

Now that you know how to keep your eyes on your target heart rate, just what kinds of activities are safe and unsafe as you prepare for the marathon of labor?

SAFE CARDIOVASCULAR SPORTS AND ACTIVITIES

Walking/Power Walking

Walking is a low-impact activity. It is inexpensive, easy, and can be done anywhere—great for women who are just starting an exercise program, during pregnancy and postpartum (postpartum workouts are suggested only *after* your doctor gives you the OK). It is also an excellent way to get outside. Try to walk briskly, using your arms to increase the intensity. Make sure your posture is good and the movement of your arms is counter to that of your legs. If you are a beginner, try walking for about ten minutes at a good pace. Over time, you'll be able to increase your time to twenty or thirty minutes. As long as you feel good, walking can be done every day. Make sure you have a comfortable pair of walking shoes. Remember, your feet widen as you get further into your pregnancy, so you may want to have a pair one half-size bigger than your normal shoe size.

Jogging/Running

Chances are, if you're a runner, you'll want to continue during pregnancy. In general, running is safe, with modifications. One piece of advice: if you have *never* been involved in a consistent running routine, now is *not* the time to start. Walking or power walking is the way to go.

Running is a great cardiovascular activity that can be done anywhere. Again, I recommend investing in a good pair of running sneakers, which should run you anywhere from $50 to $75. Go to a store that specializes in running shoes and tell the staff you're pregnant. Here, a qualified specialist can assess your size and running gait, whether you pronate or supinate, and whether your arch is high or low. Most important, they'll know that you're pregnant. Having a professional around is helpful when choosing an appropriate size for anticipated swelling in the feet.

When running while you're pregnant, it is especially important to maintain good form. Focus on your posture: your abdominals should be pulled in, your shoulders relaxed. Keep your arms close to your body. Swinging your arms wildly will only use up energy. Your hands should be close to the middle of your body. And finally, run from heel to toe with a comfortable stride length. Don't land flat-footed.

Stretching and Running

In Chapter 6, I detail stretches that should be done daily. Most likely you are aware of the importance of stretching before and after a run. If you typically don't stretch before a run, now's the time to change that routine. During pregnancy, proper stretching is more important than ever in preventing injuries and muscle soreness. I spoke about relaxin earlier, the hormone that softens and relaxes your ligaments. Since this hormone is working overtime, your ligaments and joints may be looser than normal, therefore making you more vulnerable to injury. Focus on stretching larger muscle groups first, such as the quadriceps, hamstrings, gastrocnemius (calves), and the lower back. Stretch to the point of mild discomfort.

During the first trimester, be sure to carefully monitor your heart rate. Don't overdo it. As you enter your second and third trimesters, you'll find yourself adjusting to a large belly: you are prone to falling, so be careful and try to run on flat surfaces. Most women fail to recognize that their center of gravity shifts upward during pregnancy. Eventually, you won't be able to see your feet, so this will make your workouts even trickier.

Remember, you are not training for the New York City Marathon. Modify the intensity, distance, and speed of your runs. If you feel any pain, persistent contractions, or dizziness, stop immediately and contact your doctor.

Finally, you are pregnant! You may not have the same energy as before conception. Keep that in mind and don't push yourself to exhaustion. Carry a water bottle with you; not only will it hydrate you, it will also help prevent overheating.

Swimming

One of the least dangerous of aerobic activities, swimming is a wonderful cardiovascular activity, as it improves circulation, increases muscle strength, and builds endurance.

It is safe to begin a swim program even if you weren't a swimmer before pregnancy. Be sure to stretch before and after your swim, focusing on muscles in the shoulders, upper back, and legs. If you have the energy, swim for twenty minutes (if you're a beginner this will be difficult to do), three to four times per week. Some women have found that swimming during the first trimester may help with the nausea associated with morning sickness. As you enter your second and third trimesters, don't worry about modifying your swim program, as water will protect you from overheating. I do recommend staying away from diving, especially during your third trimester.

Aerobics

Prenatal aerobic class is a great cardiovascular activity. If you are a beginner, make sure you start with a low-impact class. Be on time, as the instructor usually incorporates a warm-up, stretch, and cool-down into every class. Avoid quick changes and any movements where you could lose your balance. I like step aerobics, but I do not recommend them toward the end of the second and third trimesters.

Biking

Obviously, you want to avoid mountain biking during your pregnancy. However, using stationary (upright and recumbent) bikes and riding outdoors on smooth terrain are wonderful ways to get your heart rate up. Recumbent bikes are helpful to women who experience low-back pain, as they allow you to pedal in a reclined position.

Pilates/Yoga

Pilates is hot right now. Basically, it is a series of low-impact exercises that help develop core strength, balance, and flexibility, all of which are important to pregnant women. There are many great books and videos on Pilates as well as prenatal classes in your local gym.

ACTIVITIES TO AVOID DURING PREGNANCY

Some of these are obvious but still worth stating:

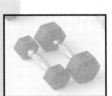

- All combat sports
- Downhill skiing
- Waterskiing
- Gymnastics
- Horseback riding
- Rough-terrain bike riding
- Step aerobics (second and third trimesters)
- Ice skating
- Scuba diving

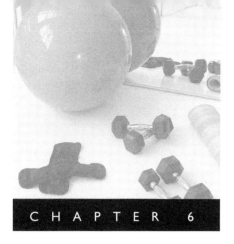

CHAPTER 6

Stretching Your Way
Through Pregnancy

I will discuss a number of stretches that you can do throughout your pregnancy. Stretching is an integral piece of any workout program and should not be neglected. Well-stretched muscles improve posture and will help ease the discomforts of labor. Be sure to warm up before doing any of the stretches. I recommend warming up with a light cardiovascular activity for about eight to ten minutes. A warm-up can be quite simple: walking, biking, or any of the cardiovascular activities I discussed earlier. You can stretch every day, throughout your pregnancy. If you experience muscular pain while stretching, you are pushing yourself too much. Stretch to the point of mild discomfort and breathe deeply. Remember, you may not be able to stay on your back for extended periods of time. If you experience any dizziness, discontinue or try stretching the same muscle group in a different position.

> ❧ *Deep, dynamic stretching should be avoided due to connective-tissue laxity. Gentle, static stretching is recommended.*

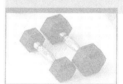

Stretches for the Lower Body

QUADRICEPS STRETCH—LYING ON YOUR SIDE

Lie down on your left side with your knees bent in front of you. Extend your left arm, resting head on outstretched arm. Grab your right ankle and gently bring your heel to your butt. Try to press your right hip forward, feeling the quadriceps stretch. Hold for fifteen seconds, then repeat with the other leg. Do each leg twice.

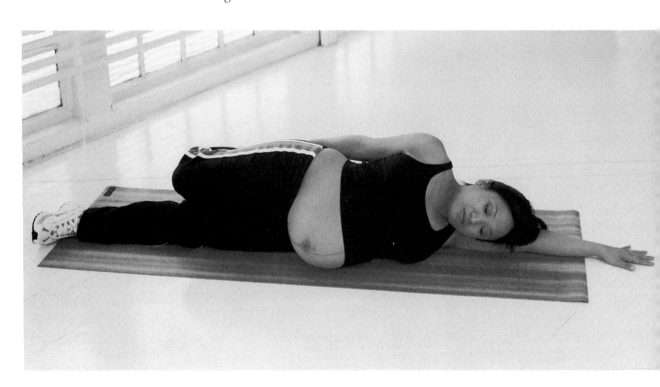

STANDING QUADRICEPS STRETCH

This stretch is more advanced. Stand up straight, being sure to maintain balance by grabbing a chair or table in front of you. Bend one leg back, holding the top of your foot. Keeping your knees together, bring your heel to your butt. Hold for fifteen seconds, then repeat with the other leg. Do each leg twice.

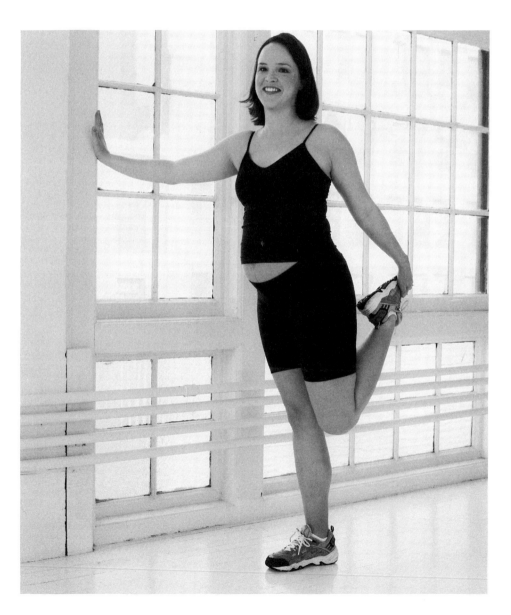

◆ *If you feel dizzy lying on your back, discontinue and try the seated hamstring stretch.*

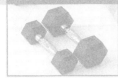

LYING HAMSTRING STRETCH

Lie flat on your back on an exercise mat or carpeted floor. Lift your left leg up perpendicular to the floor. Your right leg should be flat on the floor. Interlock your hands behind your left knee, pulling your leg to your chest. Pull to where you feel a stretch in your left hamstring. Hold for fifteen seconds, then repeat with the opposite leg.

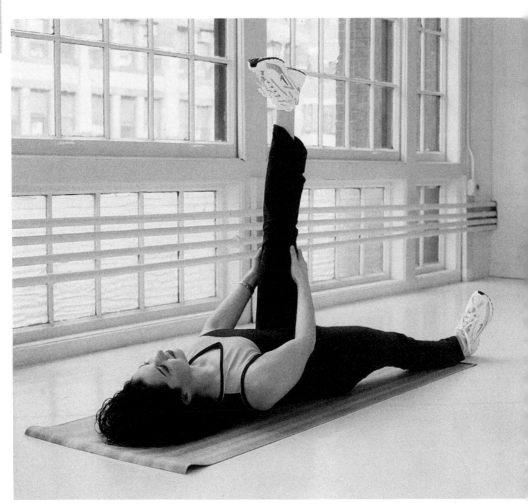

SEATED HAMSTRING STRETCH

Sit with your left leg bent, heel facing toward your right inner thigh. Keep your right leg straight. Bend forward, trying to keep your back straight. Reach toward your right foot, bringing hands forward. Hold when you feel a slight pull in the right hamstring. Repeat with opposite leg. Do each leg twice.

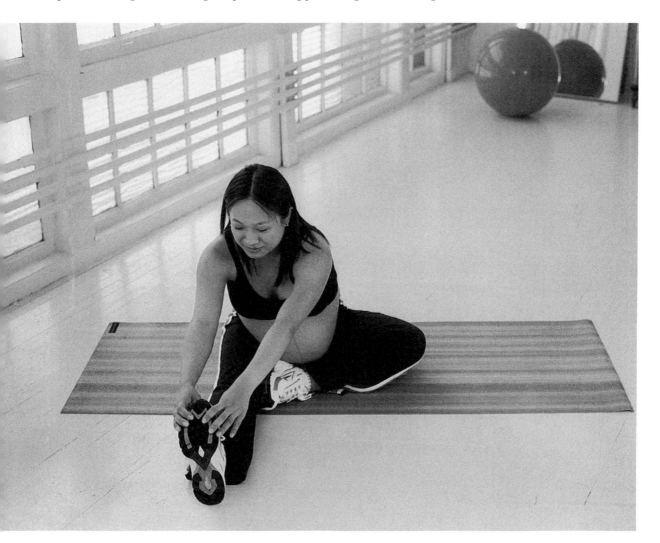

CALF STRETCH

Standing, lean forward and place both hands in front of you. Keep one leg slightly bent and step back with the other leg, pushing your heel to the ground. Try to keep your heel down to benefit from this stretch. Hold for fifteen seconds, then repeat. Do each calf twice.

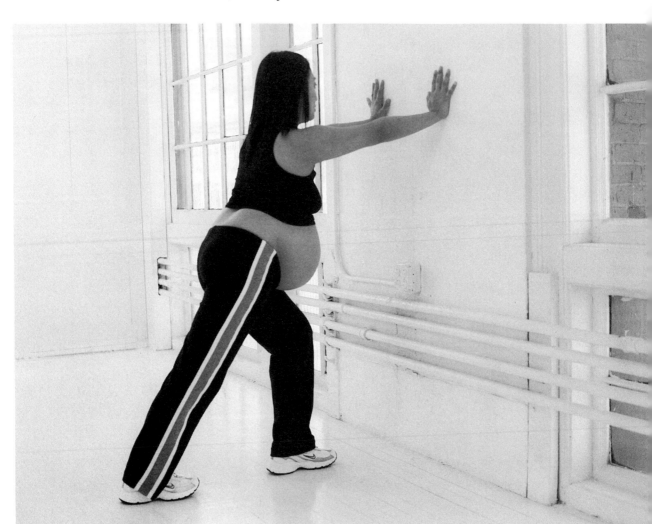

INNER THIGH STRETCH

Sitting, pull legs apart to form a comfortable V. Place your palms on the floor and gently lean forward to where you feel a slight pull in the inner thighs. Trying to keep your back straight, hold for twelve to fifteen seconds and repeat.

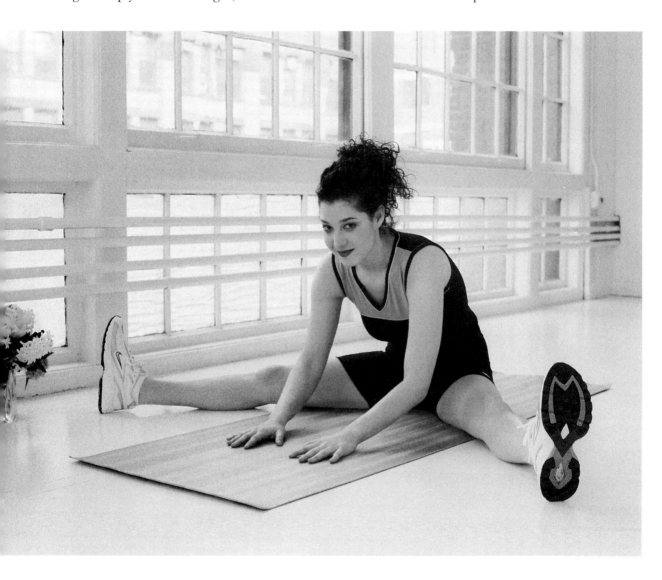

HEEL-TO-HEEL STRETCH

This is also an excellent stretch for the groin and inner thigh muscles. Sitting, place the heels of your feet together. Keep your back as straight as possible. Grab your ankles with your hands and gently press your knees down with your elbows. Hold for twelve to fifteen seconds and repeat.

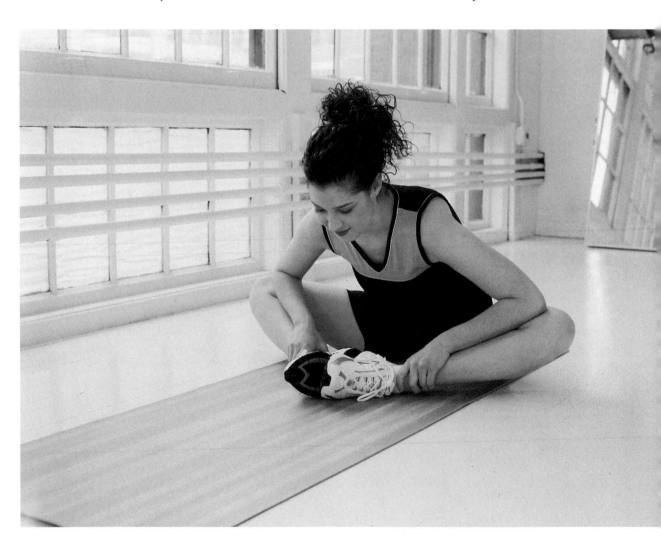

GLUTES STRETCH

Lie on your back with both feet flat on floor. Cross your left leg over your right, just above the knee. Grab your right leg behind your thigh (hamstring area) and pull both legs toward you until you feel the stretch in the left side of your glutes. Hold for ten to twelve seconds, then cross your legs the other way and stretch.

➤ If you feel any dizziness when doing this stretch, discontinue and try the sitting glute stretch.

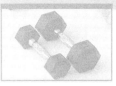

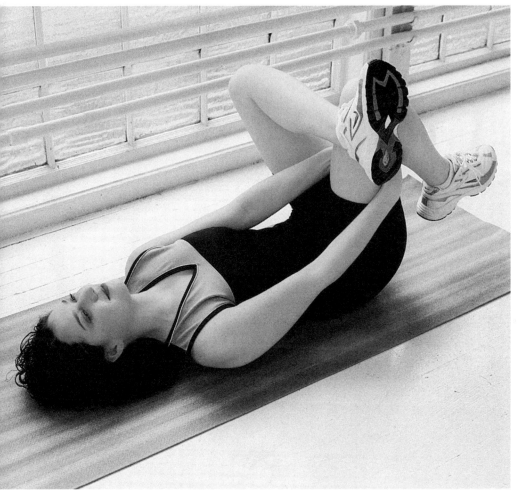

SITTING GLUTES STRETCH

Sitting, extend your left leg, toes up, keeping your back as straight as possible. Bend your right knee and place your right foot over your left knee. Gently pull your right knee into your body, feeling the stretch in your right buttock. Hold for twelve to fifteen seconds, then repeat with opposite leg. Do each leg twice.

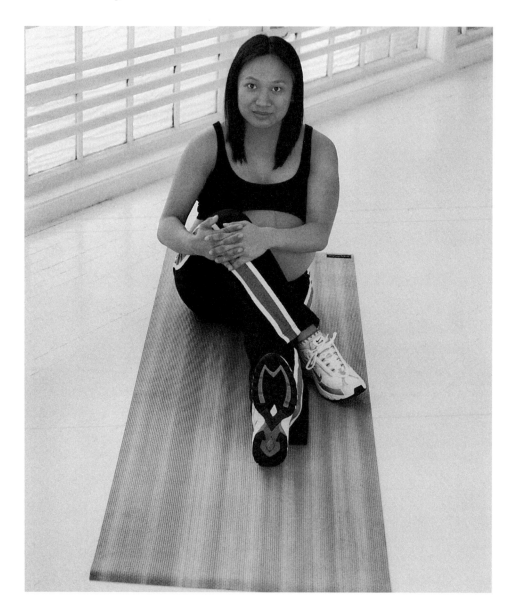

Stretches for the Lower and Upper Back

LOWER-BACK STRETCH

Spinal Twists

Sitting, cross your legs and keep your back straight. Place your right hand on your left knee and rotate, pulling your body to the left. Twist so you can comfortably look over your left shoulder. Hold ten to twelve seconds.

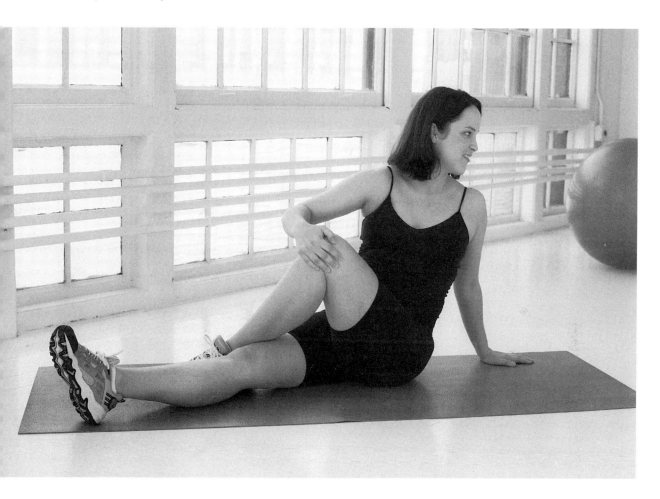

❧ *As pregnancy progresses, you can widen your knees to make this stretch more comfortable.*

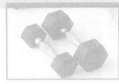

PRAYER STRETCH

Get on all fours and try to keep your butt on your heels. Keep your head face-down toward the floor. Extend your arms in front of you. Push your hips to your heels and hold for twelve to fifteen seconds.

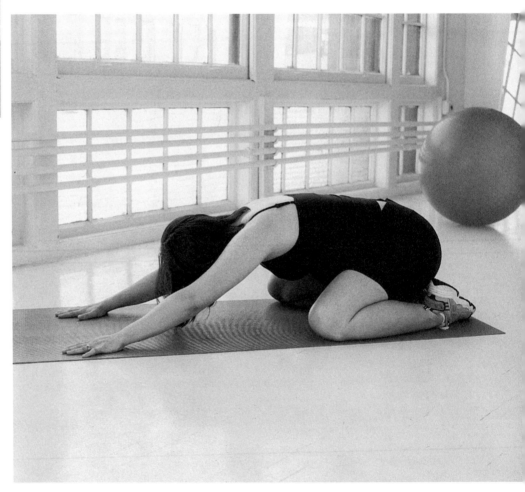

CAT STRETCH

Get on your hands and knees, keeping your back straight and relaxed. Exhale and walk your hands backward a few inches and arch your back forward into the cat pose. Hold for a count of three, inhale, and relax. Repeat three times, adding more repetitions when you feel stronger.

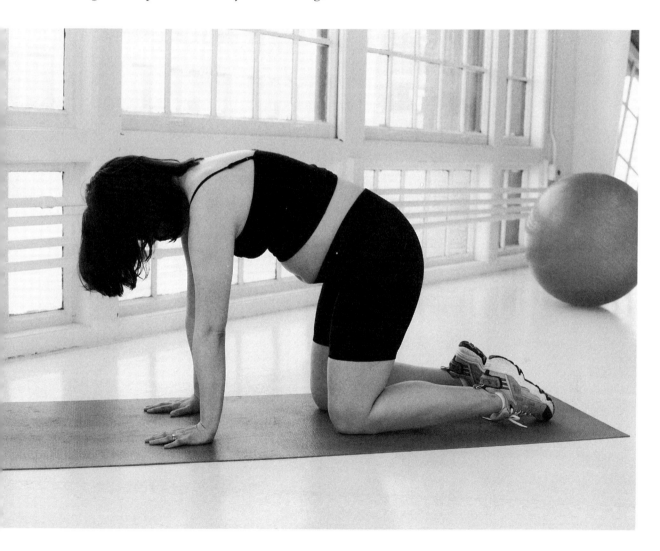

Stretches for the Upper Body

STANDING NECK STRETCH

Stand with your feet shoulder-width apart and your arms relaxed at your sides, palms facing out. Raise your right hand up toward your head and grasp the side of the crown of your head. Relax your neck and gently pull the head down so that it is leaning slightly forward and in line with your collarbone. Do not pull or push your head suddenly or stretch where you find discomfort. Hold for ten to twelve seconds, then switch hands and repeat on the other side. Do each side twice.

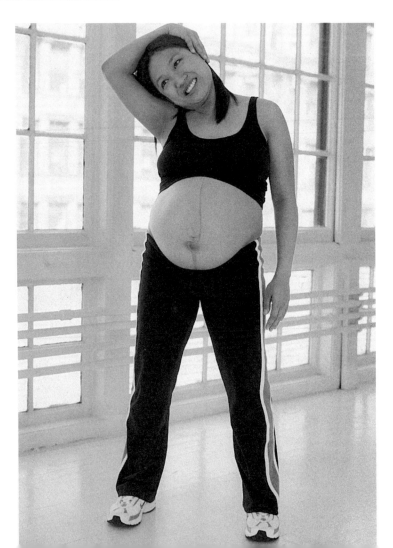

CHEST/SHOULDER STRETCH

Stand with your feet shoulder-width apart. Don't lock your knees. Clasp your hands behind your back and lift your arms behind you. Keep your back straight. Hold for twelve to fifteen seconds and repeat.

TRICEPS STRETCH

Stand with your feet shoulder-width apart. Your arms should be at your sides, palms facing backward. Raise your right arm and bring your forearm behind your head so that your elbow is at a ninety-degree angle. Bring your left hand up and over the top of your head, gently pulling the right elbow to point vertically. Hold your head against your right elbow; your right hand should rest between your shoulder blades. You should feel a stretch along your right triceps. Hold for twelve to fifteen seconds, then switch arms. Do each side twice.

(*See next page for photo.*)

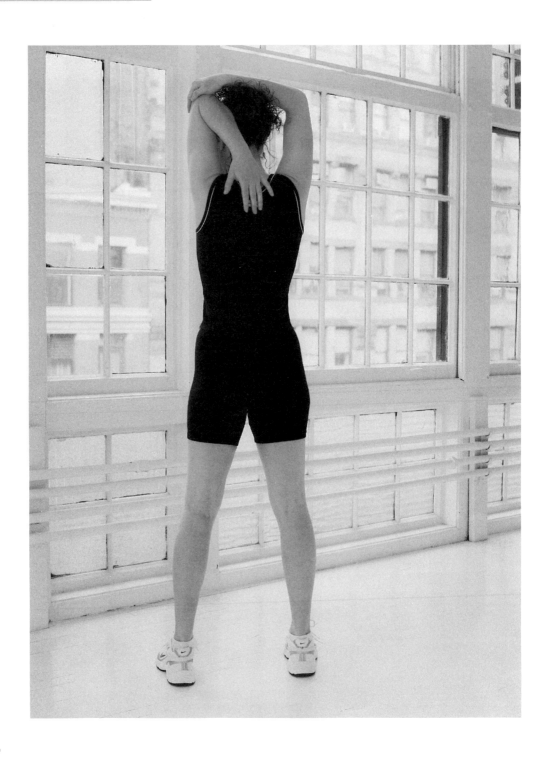

DELTOIDS/SHOULDERS STRETCH

Standing, reach your right arm across your chest, fully extended. Press your right arm into your body, pushing your right elbow with your left hand. You should feel a stretch in the back of your shoulder, or posterior deltoid. Hold for twelve to fifteen seconds, then release. Switch sides and stretch the left deltoid. Do each side twice.

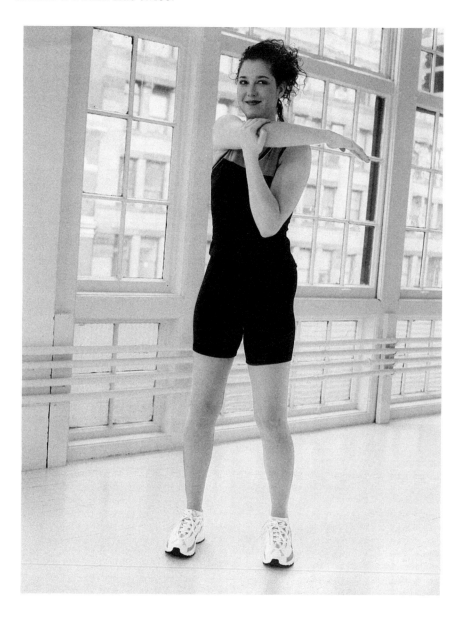

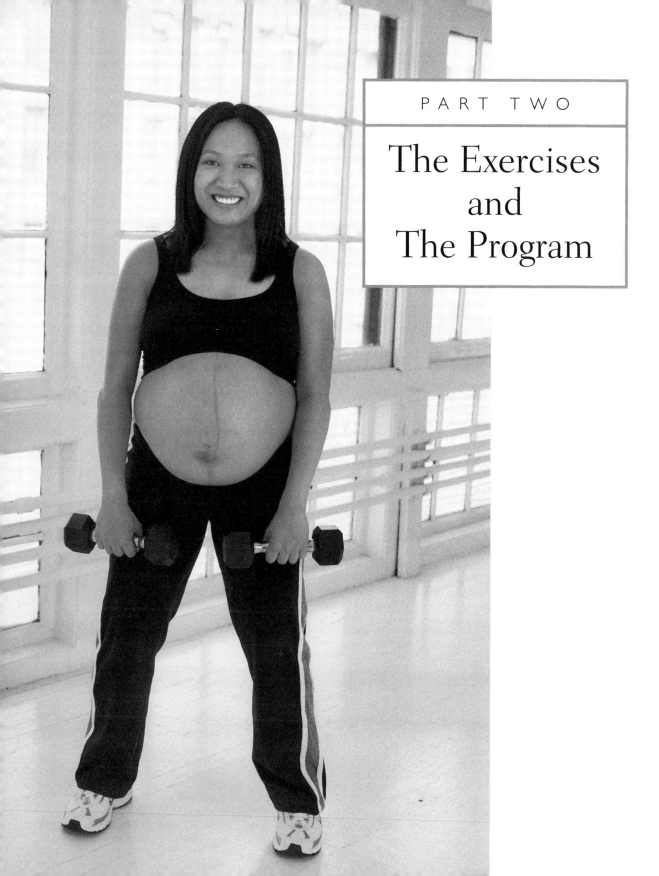

PART TWO

The Exercises and The Program

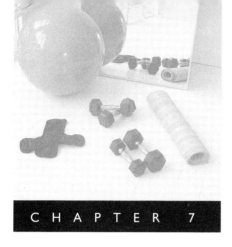

CHAPTER 7

Getting Started:
Strength Training

THE BEGINNING

Remember, if you are new to a fitness program, you want to start slow and easy. Don't try to do too much in the beginning. If you are sore and achy the day after working out, you probably did too much.

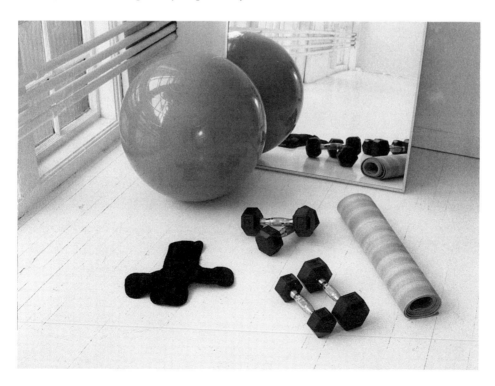

The exercises described in this chapter can be done at home and in a limited workout space. Most moms-to-be feel self-conscious in a public gym, so I devised this program to be safe, effective, and easy to do at home. Before we get started, you may want to prepare your home gym with a few pieces of equipment.

CREATING A HOME GYM:
SIMPLE ITEMS YOU WILL NEED TO BEGIN YOUR BUFF MOM'S WORKOUT

There are countless numbers of gadgets you can purchase when creating a home gym. Spending hundreds of dollars is not only a waste of money but totally unnecessary. Getting the job done requires commitment, not a lot of money.

Dumbbells

Dumbbells come in various shapes, sizes, and colors. They also come in various prices. Time and time again I tell my clients that a $10 set of five-pound dumbbells weighs the same as a $25 set of five-pound dumbbells. They both do the same job.

Depending on your level of strength, start off with three to four sets of dumbbells, increasing in weight. Beginners should start off with three-, five-, and eight-pound dumbbells. Intermediate and more advanced moms-to-be should start off with heavier weights (five-, ten-, and twelve-pound dumbbells). People often ask what's best for optimum results: free weights or machines? Machines make things easier for you, in a way. They direct your movement patterns. Free weights force you to strengthen any imbalance you have. They allow you to train each muscle group separately; your dominant side can't do all the work. Sometimes, when using machines, your dominant or stronger side will compensate for your weaker side when you start to get tired.

Fitness Ball

A fitness ball is an excellent addition to your home gym. Traditionally, fitness balls were used by rehabilitation and physical-therapy patients. Today, they can be found in almost any gym. Fitness balls work on the concept of core strength and balance. The core muscle group are the muscles of the abdominals and lower back, hips, and spine. When you're pregnant, it is especially important to strengthen these two areas. Most people have incredibly weak core strength. They release their abs or arch their back when performing a specific exercise. What they're actually doing is compensating by using different parts of their body to do the desired strengthening exercise. This is common; I see it all the time in public gyms and when my clients perform abdominal exercises. To make up for their lack of strength, many people use their hip flexor muscles, not their abdominal muscles. The fitness ball strengthens the abdominals through a full range of motion without using the hip flexor muscles.

Core strength and balance are important in developing and improving overall muscular strength. The fitness ball is especially useful for pregnant women, as it supports the back and abdominal muscles during the exercises. Just draping yourself over the ball, facedown, will relieve some of the aches and pains of the lower back during pregnancy and labor.

A fitness ball usually comes with a pump. This allows you to inflate and deflate it for easy storage. It also comes in various sizes. When purchasing one, make sure you buy a ball according to your height. Inflate the ball so it's pretty firm. If your ball is not inflated enough, you will sink into the ball and risk losing a safe body position. With a growing belly, your center of gravity changes during pregnancy. Make sure you adapt and shift your body accordingly.

Exercise Mats

Exercise mats are important, especially if you don't have a soft, carpeted area to work out on. Mats are usually inexpensive and easy to find in any sporting equipment or department store.

Ankle Weights

As you progress through the lower-body exercises, I recommend using ankle weights to intensify your workout. They are worn around the ankle, usually attached by Velcro. Ankle weights are relatively inexpensive, about $15 to $25.

Bench/Step

A bench or step is useful not only for toning muscles of the lower body but also for providing a good cardiovascular workout. Lengths and heights vary. Most steps have adjustable risers; the higher the step, the more intense the workout.

Mirror

A full-length mirror will help you keep your form in check. Proper form is essential when you're pregnant.

Favorite CD

This is the time to have fun. Go out and buy your favorite CD. Nothing gets you going like good music when you're working out.

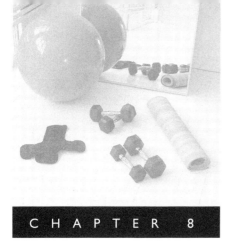

CHAPTER 8

The Exercises:
Keeping That Great Body and
Preparing for Labor

The following chapter will guide you through a series of upper-body, lower-body, and abdominal strength-training exercises all geared toward the mom-to-be. (Make sure you are integrating cardiovascular fitness and stretching into your program for optimum results.) These exercises have proven successful for the countless number of pregnant women I have trained. When you're doing them, make sure you drink plenty of water. Not only is it good for you, but, as I've mentioned before, it cools you down. Since your core temperature is a bit higher during pregnancy, you want to be especially conscious of not overheating your body.

Kegel Exercises

Kegel exercises—named after Dr. Arnold Kegel, a Los Angeles gynecologist, in the mid-1940s—were originally developed as a method of controlling incontinence in women following childbirth. The principle behind Kegel exercises is to strengthen the muscles of the pelvic floor, thereby improving the urethral and rectal sphincter function. Kegel exercises are now recommended during pregnancy to strengthen the muscles of the pelvic floor, which support the urethra, bladder, uterus, and rectum, and can weaken due to the excess weight of the baby and fluid. Kegel exercises can and should be done daily to strengthen the muscles.

- Tighten and relax these muscles over and over, holding for ten seconds, then releasing. Repeat fifteen to twenty-five times, four to five times per day.
- Squeeze the pelvic-floor muscles, as if you're trying to stop the flow of urine (but not during the act of urinating).

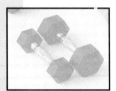

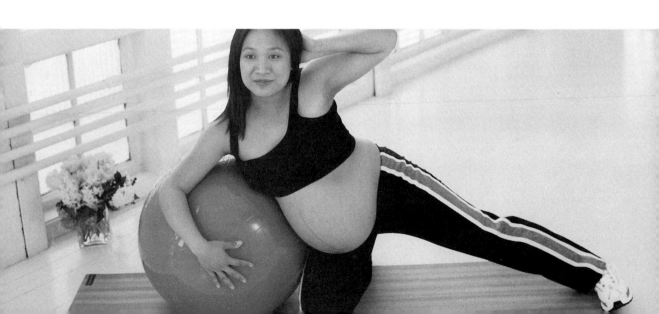

OTHER KEGEL VARIATIONS

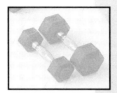

- Hold for five seconds, then relax, twelve to fifteen times. Don't overdo it.
- While sitting in a chair, keep your feet slightly apart and your back straight. Tighten and relax your pelvic-floor muscles, holding for five seconds, then releasing.
- While sitting on the floor, keep your back flat against a wall. Keep your feet slightly apart. To the count of five, gradually tighten your pelvic-floor muscles, increasing tension with each count. Slowly release, to the count of five, to the starting position.

Kegeling provides many benefits:

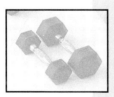

- Conditioned muscles will make birth easier, and your perineum will more likely remain intact (with fewer tears and episiotomies).
- Sexual enjoyment is enhanced for both partners.
- Kegeling can prevent prolapses of pelvic organs.
- Kegeling can help prevent incontinence when you sneeze or cough.

THE WEIGHTS FACTOR . . .

All of the outlined exercises are geared toward maintaining strength and flexibility during pregnancy. By no means are they designed to put excessive strain on your body. You should feel comfortable, without overexerting yourself, when weight training. You will need to avoid using heavy weights and assuming certain positions. If you take the necessary precautions and have good technique, weight training is a great way to tone and strengthen your muscles and prepare yourself for labor.

You should be able to do eight to twelve repetitions of a particular exercise with good form. Your last repetition should be challenging, but remember: when you're pregnant, you are not trying to break any records. Start with one set of each exercise and work up to a second set (especially true for beginners). Proper form is mandatory! Abdominal strengthening should always be done last in your workout. Also, avoid working out the same muscle group two days in a row.

If you decide to do a strength-training program on a different day than your cardio workout, it's important to incorporate a warm-up and cool-down into each session. I recommend a warm-up of five to ten minutes before lifting any weights. Not only will this help you avoid injury, but your muscles need to be ready for work. Warm-ups can include any of the cardiovascular activities I described in Chapter 5, as well as stretches for the chest, legs, arms, back, and shoulders. A proper cool-down should always include stretching (Chapter 6).

Other than avoiding exercising on your back for extended periods of time, modifications to your weight-training program depend on how you feel physically. As I stated earlier, your center of gravity changes as your pregnancy progresses. Be conscious of this and make modifications if necessary. You may have to decrease the weights and repetitions as you get bigger. Listen to what your body is telling you. Later in pregnancy, you may experience Braxton Hicks contractions. This tightening of the lower abdomen is common. If it occurs, stop what you're doing and wait for the contractions to ease. If they are persistent, make sure to bring them to the attention of your doctor.

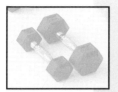

- *Repetition:* doing the movement one time. Most of the time you will be instructed to do a given number of repetitions. This means you are to do the same movement "X" times without resting in between.
- *Set:* a completion of a series of repetitions. If you are instructed to do two sets, you may rest in between for a minute or so.

Unless otherwise stated, each concentric (weight brought toward your body) and eccentric (weight moved away from your body) phase should be done to a count of four. Make sure to exhale on the eccentric phase, inhaling on the concentric phase. If you can do one set comfortably, go ahead and do a second set.

Exercises that require you to lie on your back are probably best avoided after twenty weeks into pregnancy, since lying this way may limit blood flow to your uterus and baby.

Continue doing the exercises that feel comfortable, but don't strain yourself by attempting new, unfamiliar lifts or by using too much resistance. Exercises that mimic your daily activities, like step-ups, split squats, and mini-lunges, are best. Here are some tips to keep in mind:

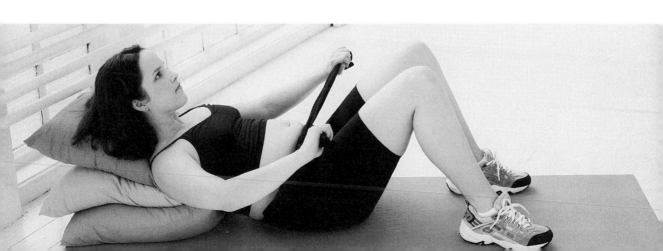

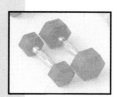

- Try to work the larger muscle groups before working the smaller ones.
- Squats are good, but never bend your knees more than ninety degrees. Slower is better, and the fitness ball is a great tool for keeping good form.
- For your abs, cut out traditional sit-ups and focus on gaining control of your lower abdominals. Sitting on a fitness ball and doing Kegel exercises will help.

THE BUFF MOM-TO-BE CHECKLIST

OK, you're almost ready to go. Make sure you go over the following checklist to ensure a safe and effective Buff Mom-to-be program:

Permission from your doctor. Go over the desired exercise program and make sure it's safe for you.

Commit yourself. Working out once a week is OK but not great. For optimum results, try to aim for three times per week.

Comfort! Wear workout clothes that are comfortable. Gear should be able to "breathe," ensuring that you don't overheat.

Did you warm up? Cool down? Stretch?

Keep an eye on your heart rate.

Breathe appropriately. When working on your cardiovascular fitness, make sure to breathe in through the nose and exhale from your mouth. When strength training, exhale on the exertion, inhale on the down phase.

How are your abdominals doing? Keep checking throughout your pregnancy to see if you have a diastasis. Diastasis is a separation of the two halves of the rectus abdominus along the middle of your belly. This is common during pregnancy. See page 87 for a complete explanation of a diastasis.

Have water nearby.

Strengthening and Toning the Upper Body

Don't feel as if you have to do all of these in one day. Pick out a few, add some cardio before or after, and mix it up! Most of all . . . *have fun!*

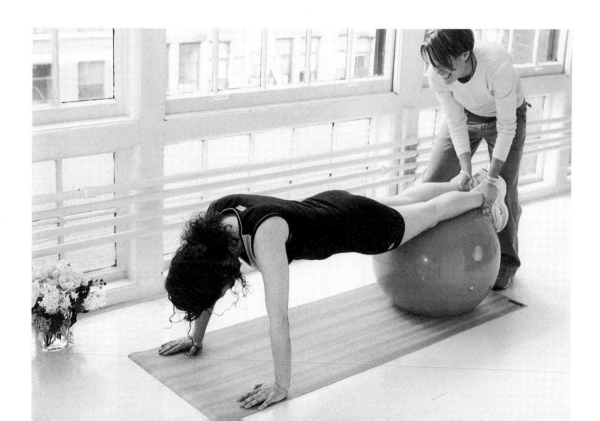

MODIFIED PUSH-UPS

From a kneeling position, place your hands flat on the ground, shoulder-width apart. Inch your hands forward so they are in front of you. To the count of four, bend your elbows and lower your chest to the floor. Keep your head steady, looking straight down toward the floor. Return to the starting position to the count of four. To increase the intensity of the exercise, lift one knee off the ground, keeping your weight balanced on one knee and your hands.

Do two sets of eight to ten repetitions.

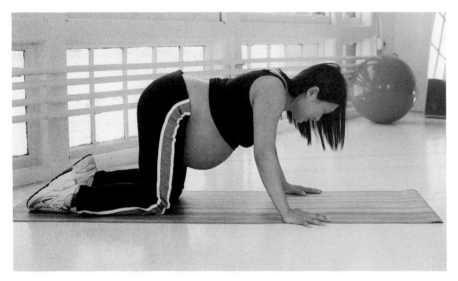

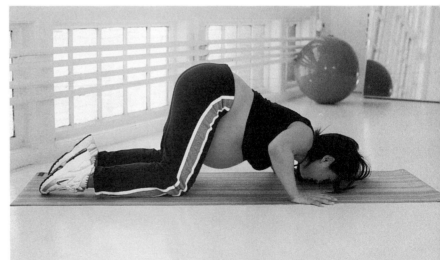

PUSH-UPS WITH BALL

From a kneeling position, pull a fitness ball in toward your quads, drape your torso over it, and put your hands on the floor in front of it. Tighten abs and walk hands forward until your hips are in front of the ball and your back is flat. Your feet will not be on the floor. This is the plank position. Continue to tighten your abs, letting the ball roll slightly under you toward your knees. Hold this position.

To the count of four, bend your elbows and lower your chest to the floor. Don't place your hands too wide or too narrow, and don't lead with your hips. Inhale as you lower your chest to the ball; exhale as you return to the starting position.

You can increase the intensity of the exercise by placing the ball closer to your feet. Placing the ball more toward the midline of your body will make the exercise easier.

Do two sets of eight to ten repetitions; recommended only for first and second trimesters.

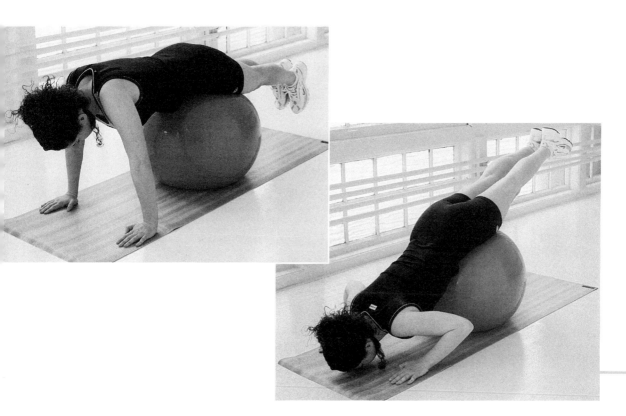

CHEST PRESS WITH BALL

Lie back on a fitness ball so your head and neck are stabilized. Push your hips up, and keep your abdominal and butt muscles tight. Pick up a dumbbell in each hand and hold them above you, with your palms facing out. Keep the dumbbells shoulder-width apart. Don't allow your hips to drop. To the count of four, slowly lower the dumbbells until they are even with your chest. Raise them to the starting position, same tempo. Make sure to exhale on the exertion and breathe in when lowering.

Do two sets of eight to twelve repetitions.

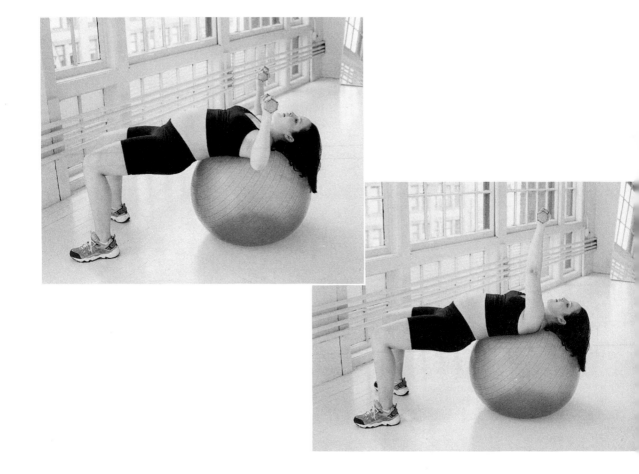

OVERHEAD PRESS ON BALL

Sit squarely on a fitness ball, feet flat on the floor. Maintain a flat back by keeping your abdominals tight. Hold two dumbbells just in front of your shoulders, palms facing out. Look straight ahead, keeping your head steady. Extend your arms and lift the dumbbells over your head. The dumbbells should almost touch each other at the extension. Pause and lower the dumbbells to your shoulders. Envision making a triangle from start to finish. Don't lock your elbows or arch your back.

Do two sets of eight to ten repetitions.

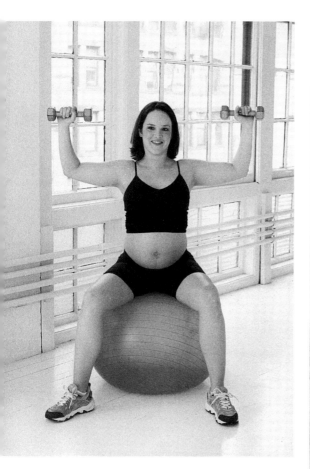

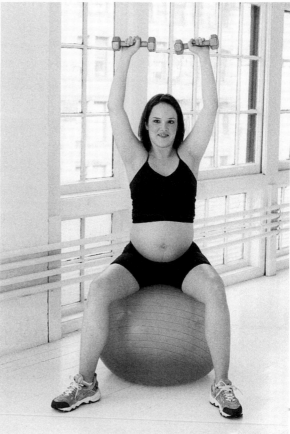

ALTERNATING ARM RAISES

Standing, hold a dumbbell in each hand, palms facing your body and resting on your thighs. Keep your knees slightly bent, feet shoulder-width apart. With your right arm, slowly raise the dumbbell to shoulder height. Pause, then lower to starting position. Repeat, alternating arms.

Do two sets of eight to ten repetitions.

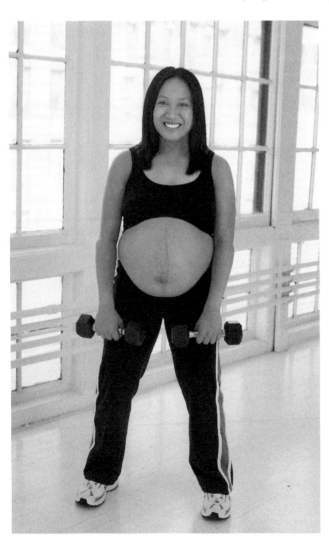 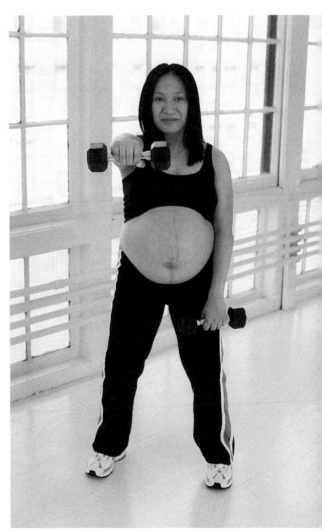

UPWARD ROWS

Stand with straight back and soft knees, feet shoulder-width apart. With a dumbbell in each hand, lift the weights up toward your chin. Keep the weight close to the body, and avoid arching the back and swinging the arms. The elbows need to stay above the dumbbells, raised no higher than your shoulders.

Do two sets of eight to ten repetitions.

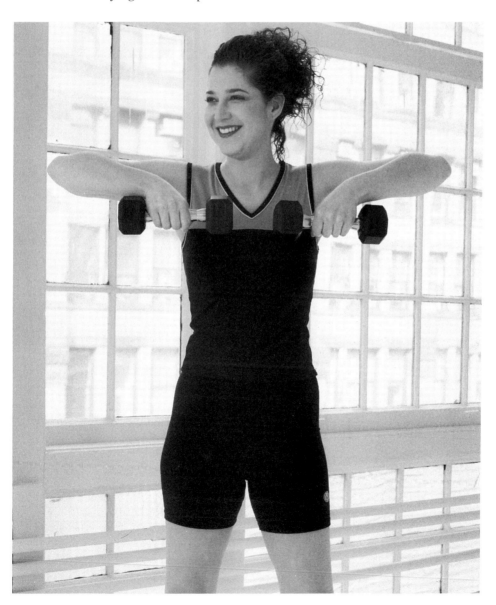

FLIES—LATERAL RAISE

Standing, hold a dumbbell in each hand, palms facing in. Be sure to keep your back straight, knees soft. With your arms bent approximately ninety degrees, raise the weights to shoulder height. Avoid rocking your body. Keeping your abdominals and glutes tight will prevent arching of your back. Pause, then slowly lower to starting position.

Do two sets of eight to ten repetitions.

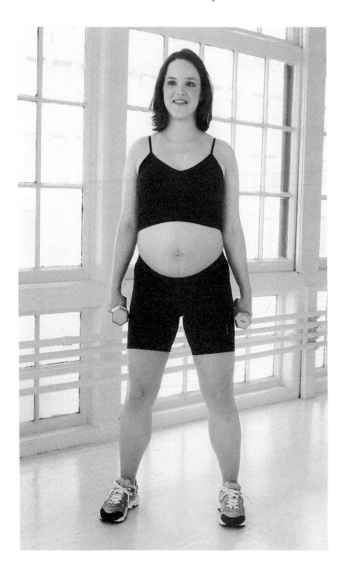 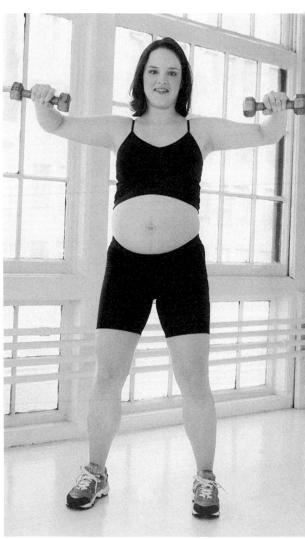

CONCENTRATION CURL ON BALL

Sit on a fitness ball, knees bent and shoulder-width apart. Holding a dumbbell in your right hand, lean forward, placing the back of the right upper arm inside your right thigh. Your right palm should be facing your left leg, left hand on top of left knee for support. While keeping your abdominals tight, bring dumbbell toward your right shoulder, wrist locked. Slowly lower to starting position.

Do two sets of eight to ten repetitions.

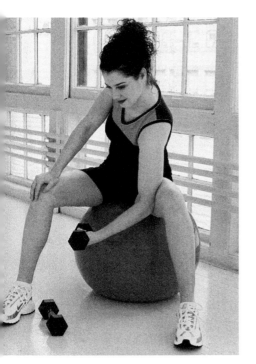

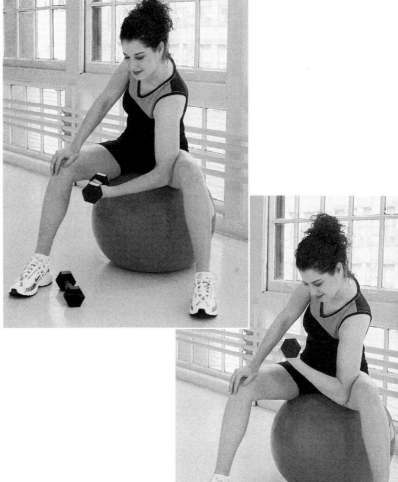

ALTERNATING BICEPS CURL

Standing, hold a dumbbell in each hand, arms extended at your sides, palms facing in. Keep your back straight and your feet shoulder-width apart. Slowly curl the right dumbbell up toward your right biceps, slowly turning your wrist so your palm is facing in. Aim to keep your elbows tucked into your sides, and avoid swinging the weights up or arching your back. Lower to the starting position, turning your wrist so your palm is facing in at the end of the curl. Be sure to keep your butt and abdominals tight throughout the movement. Repeat with the left arm.

Do two sets of ten to twelve repetitions.

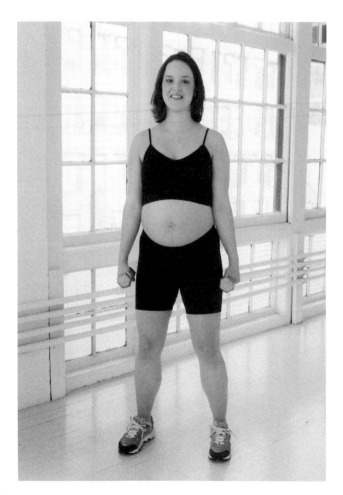
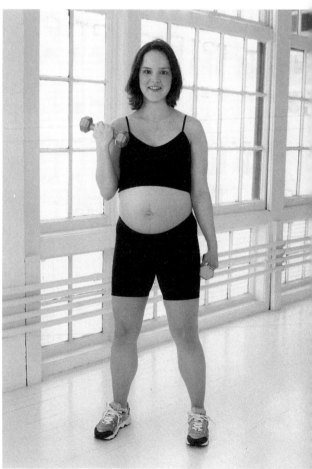

HAMMER CURLS ON BALL

Sitting on a fitness ball, keep your knees shoulder-width apart, feet flat on the floor. Hold a dumbbell in each hand, arms extended, palms facing in. With the right hand, bring the dumbbell up to your right shoulder, making sure to keep your right elbow tucked into your side. Slowly lower, then repeat with left arm. Be sure to keep your back straight and abdominals tight throughout the movement.

Do two sets of ten to twelve repetitions.

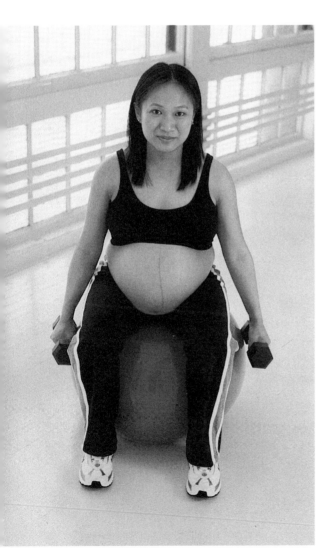
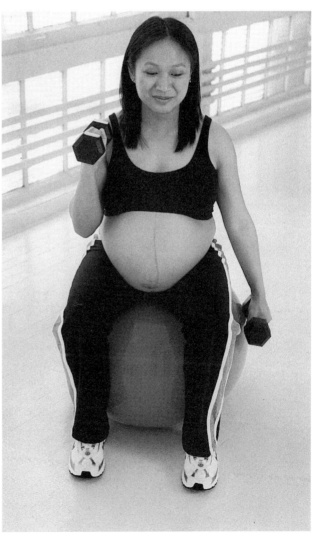

TRICEPS EXTENSION—OVERHEAD

Sitting on a fitness ball or bench, keep your knees bent, feet flat on the floor. Holding one dumbbell, bring it behind your head, keeping your elbow close to your ear. With your abdominals tight, slowly straighten your arm to full extension, being careful to keep elbow soft (not locking). Lower to starting position and repeat.

Do two sets of eight to ten repetitions with each arm.

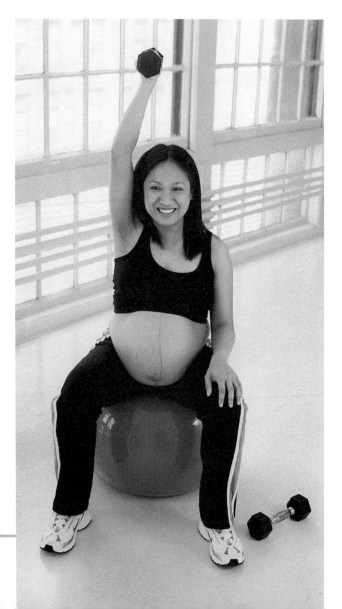
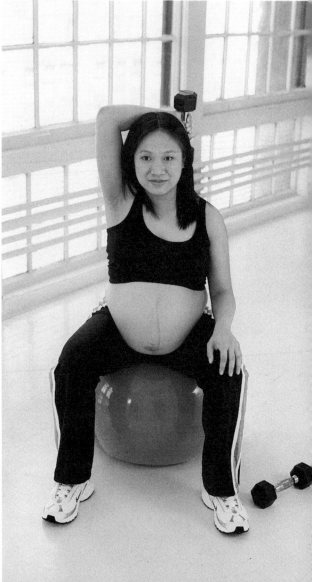

TRICEPS EXTENSION ON BALL

Lie on a fitness ball, placing it behind your head so that your head and neck are stabilized. Your knees should be shoulder-width apart, feet flat on the floor. With a dumbbell in each hand, palms facing in, push your hips up, squeezing your butt and keeping your abdominals contracted. Bend your elbows and place dumbbells next to each ear. Slowly extend your arms straight above, being careful not to lock them. Slowly lower them to starting position and repeat.

This exercise strengthens not only the triceps muscle but also the abdominals and muscles of the lower back. As pregnancy progresses, be careful of your center of gravity and balance when doing this exercise.

Do two sets of eight to ten repetitions.

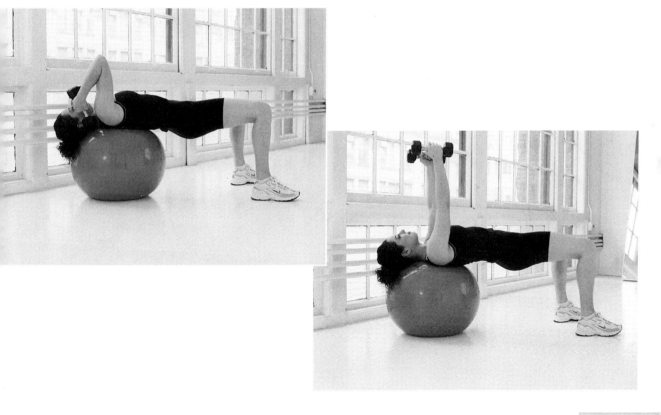

TRICEPS DIPS

Sit on a bench or sturdy chair, your hands gripping the front edge of the seat. Your legs should be bent with your feet flat on the floor. With your legs together, move forward until your hips and butt are off the seat. Slowly lower your butt toward the floor, keeping your abdominals tight and your elbows pointing behind you. A common mistake is to allow your elbows to go to the sides. Once your arms are bent at a ninety-degree angle, slowly raise your body to the starting position, arms fully extended and elbows soft.

This exercise is recommended during the first and early second trimester. *Do two sets of eight repetitions.*

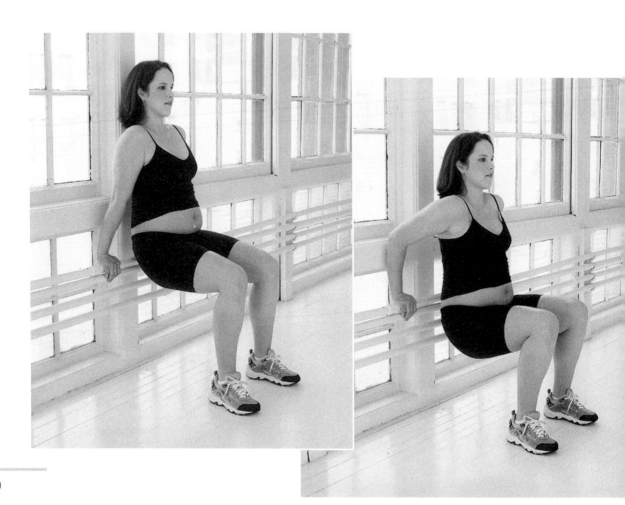

ONE-ARM TRICEPS KICKBACKS

Place your right knee in the middle of a bench or sturdy chair. Your right hand should be flat on the bench, palm in line with shoulder, for added support. Your left leg should be extended behind you. Keeping your left elbow tucked in and close to your body, palm facing in, extend a dumbbell back and away from your body until your arm is straight and parallel to the floor. Pause, tightening your triceps, then return to the starting position. Keep your back flat and head straight, focusing on the floor.

Do two sets of eight to ten repetitions.

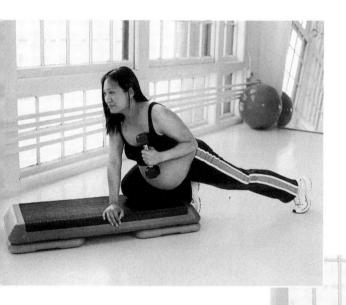

Strengthening and Toning the Lower Body

Pick out a few of these great lower-body workouts and add them to your upper-body routine.

LEG CURL WITH BALL

Lie on your back with a fitness ball under your heels and the lower portion of your legs. Your arms should be at your sides, palms facing down. Lift your hips/pelvis up as high as you can. Try to keep your weight on your upper back and shoulders. Slowly, roll the ball toward your butt, using your heels and lower legs. Once the ball is almost touching your butt, return to the starting position. Don't drop your hips throughout the set.

Do two sets of eight to ten repetitions.

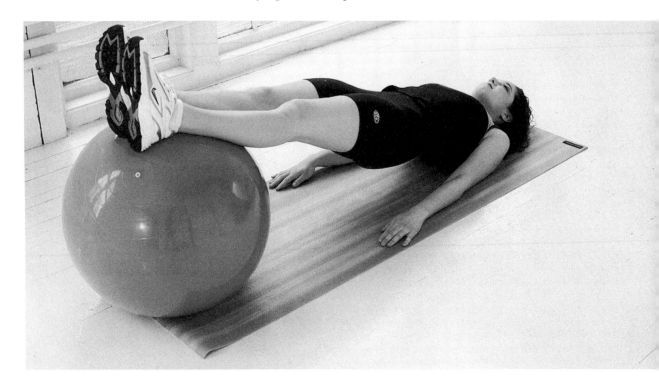

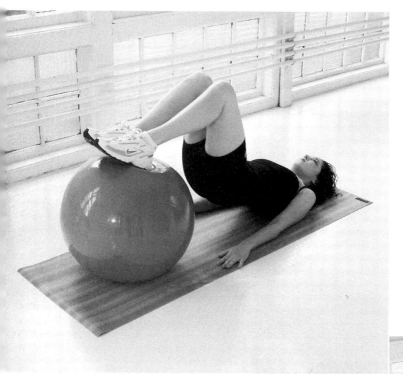

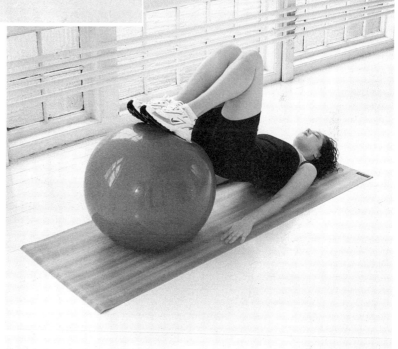

DUMBBELL SQUATS

Hold a five-to-ten-pound dumbbell (depending on your strength and ability) between your knees. Slighty pronate (turn out) your feet. Keeping your elbows slightly bent, lower your body, bending at the knees until your thighs are parallel to the floor. Be sure to keep your back straight, head looking straight ahead. Return to the starting position to the count of four.

Do two sets of eight to twelve repetitions.

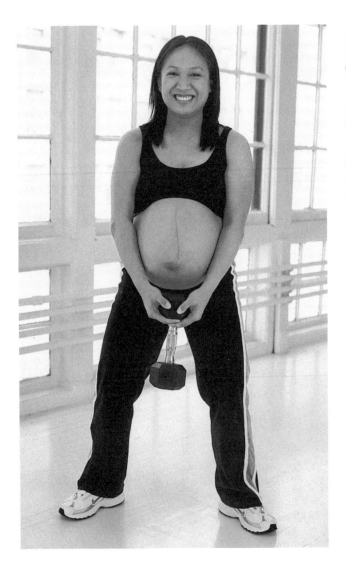

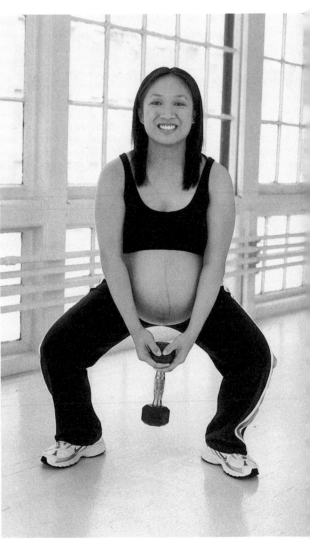

STEP-UPS WITH BENCH

Placing a workout step or bench about a foot in front of you, hold a dumbbell in each hand, arms hanging by your sides, palms facing in. (As you progress in your pregnancy, dumbbells may not be necessary as your own body weight increases.) Feet should be shoulder-width apart, knees soft. Leading with the right foot, step up onto the bench, placing foot squarely and firmly on the surface. As you step up, try to contract the quadriceps muscle on the right leg.

Do two sets of eight to twelve repetitions.

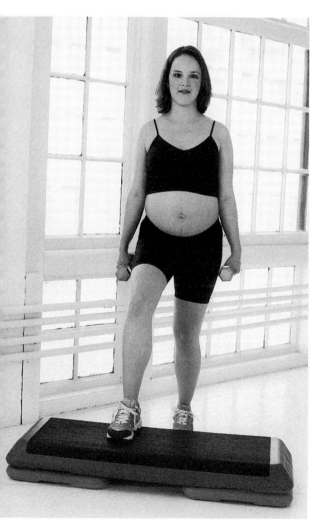
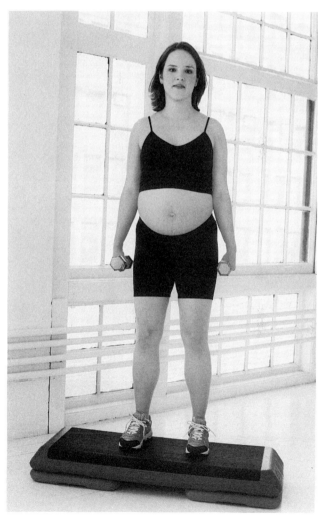

WALL SITS WITH BALL

Place a fitness ball between your lower back and a wall. Hold a dumbbell in each hand, arms hanging by your side, palms facing in. (As you progress in your pregnancy, dumbbells may not be necessary as your own body weight increases.) Keeping your lower back against the ball, walk your feet forward about two feet, and keep your feet shoulder-width apart. Keeping back straight, shoulders back, and chest out, to a count of four, slowly bend your knees to a ninety-degree angle. Your knees should stay over your toes. Pushing through the heels, slowly return to starting position to a count of four.

Do ten times, rest, then repeat.

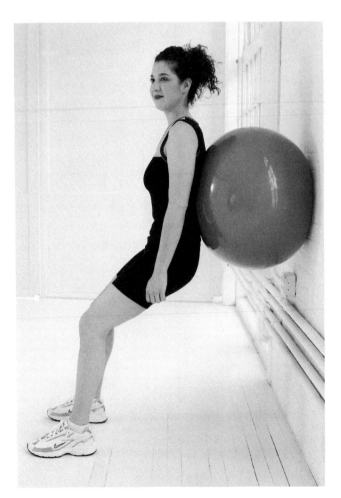
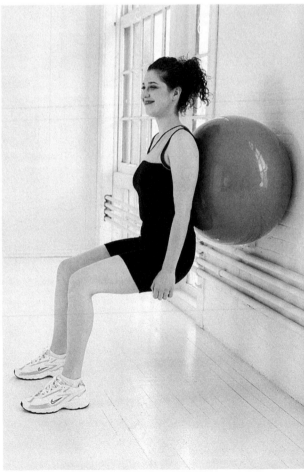

ALTERNATING QUADRICEPS LUNGES

Standing, hold two dumbbells in each hand, palms facing in and arms at your sides. (As your pregnancy progresses, dumbbells may not be necessary.) Your feet should be shoulder-width apart and your abdominals tight. With your left foot, take a step forward. Your right leg should be almost straight. Slowly lower your body by bending your left leg. Be sure to keep the left knee over the left toe when lowering. Just before your right knee touches the ground, slowly push up to the starting position. Repeat, switching legs.

Due to a shift in your center of gravity, it may be helpful to grasp a chair or doorknob for added balance.

Do two sets of eight to ten repetitions.

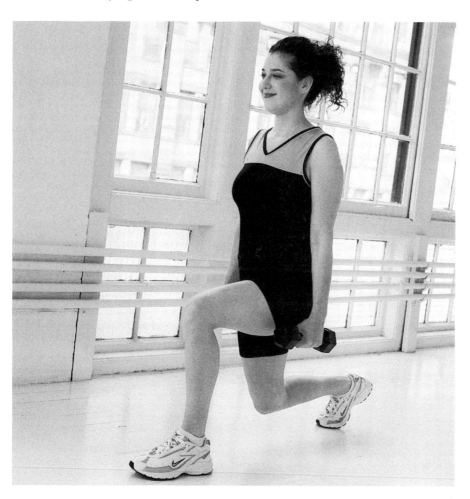

BUTT LIFTS WITH BALL

Lie on an exercise mat or carpeted floor. Place your feet on a fitness ball, slightly apart. Your toes should be pointed toward the ceiling, your arms at your sides, palms down. Lift your hips toward the ceiling, squeezing your butt and contracting your abdominals at the same time. Pause, then slowly lower until your butt almost touches the ground.

Do two sets of ten to twelve repetitions.

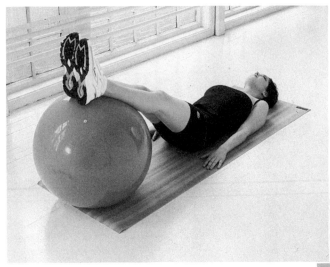

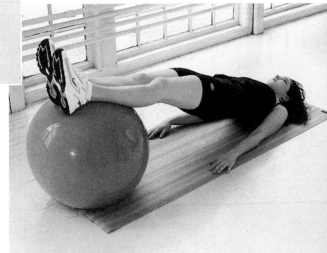

KNEELING LEG LIFT

Kneel with forearms and knees on the floor, back flat and head steady, looking toward the floor. Keep your abdominals tight. Lift your left leg behind you, bending your knee at a ninety-degree angle. Push your left foot as high as it can go, keeping the bottom of your foot facing the ceiling. Lower leg back to the ninety-degree-angle position. Repeat; after one set, switch legs. For added resistance, use a light ankle weight.

Do two sets of twelve to fifteen repetitions.

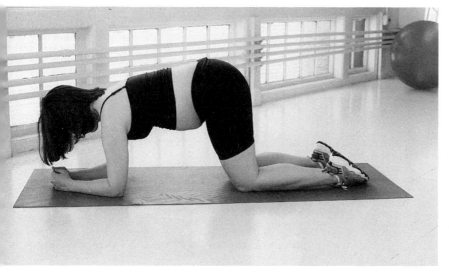

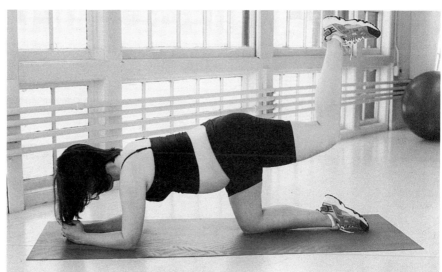

CALF RAISES OFF STEP

Standing on a bench or step (at least five inches high), face a wall or sturdy object for support. Your feet should be shoulder-width apart, legs straight. Let your heels drop slightly off the surface of the step until you feel a slight stretch in your calves. Lift up onto the balls of your feet and toes. Slowly lower and repeat.

Do two sets of ten to twelve repetitions.

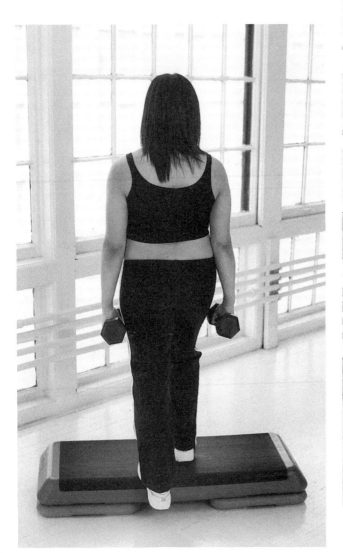

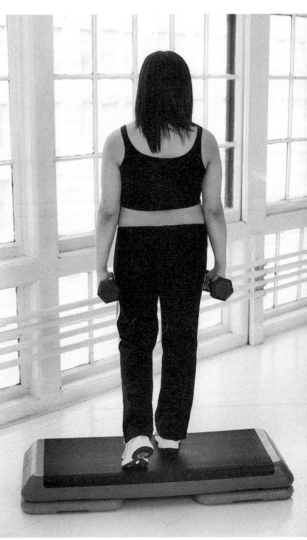

SIDE LEG LIFT

Lie on your left side and cross your upper leg (right) over your lower leg (left), and rest your right foot on the floor. Raise your left leg a few inches off the floor, up toward the ceiling, then lower again, aiming to keep your left foot off the floor at all times throughout the exercise. Try to keep the knee and toes of your right leg facing forward. Light ankle weights will make this exercise more challenging.

Do two sets of eight to ten repetitions.

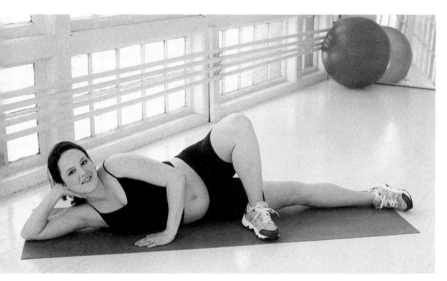

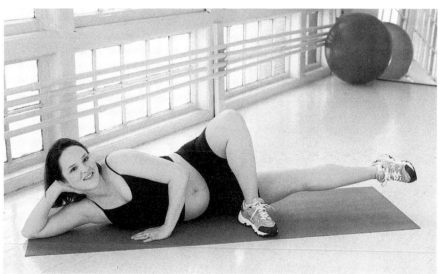

ADDUCTOR SQUEEZE WITH PILLOW

Sitting on a fitness ball, place a firm pillow between your knees and keep your feet flat on the floor. Keeping your abdominals tight and back straight, bring your knees together, squeezing the pillow with your knees. Pause and return to the starting position, keeping pillow steady and not letting it drop to the ground.

Do two sets of ten to twelve repetitions.

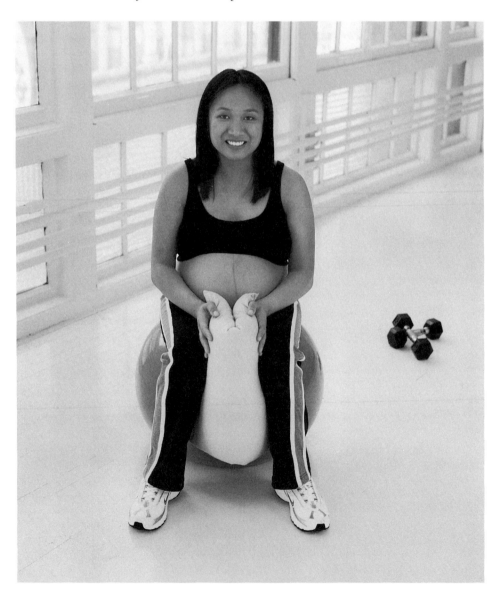

ABDUCTOR LEG LIFT

Lie on a mat or carpeted surface, on your right side, resting your head comfortably on one hand or on your upper arm. Keeping your knees and toes pointing forward, smoothly lift your left leg forty-five degrees. You can bend your right leg and use your arms to aid balance. Slowly lower and repeat for one set. Switch legs and repeat. Ankle weights can be used to make this exercise more challenging.

Do two sets of ten to twelve repetitions.

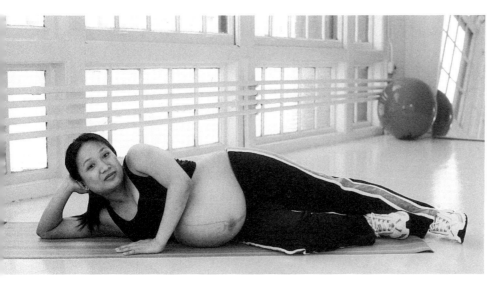

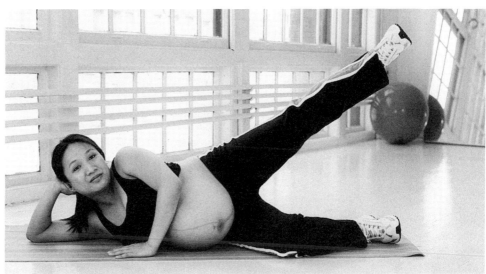

Must–Do Exercises for the Back

The following exercises are designed to help relieve the discomfort you may feel as your back tries to support the baby growing inside you. They help to strengthen and stretch the muscles of the back, hips, and abdomen.

PELVIC LIFTS

Lie on your back with your knees bent and your feet flat on the floor. Inhale and allow your abdomen to expand. Exhale and lift your tailbone toward your navel, keeping your hips on the floor. At the top of the tilt, tighten your buttocks, then release.

Do two sets of eight to ten repetitions.

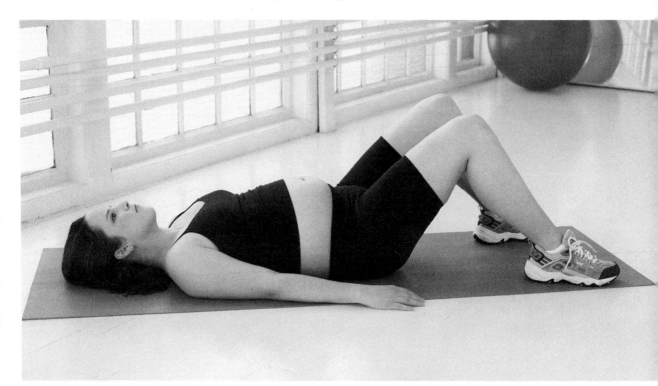

PELVIC TILTS

Lie on your back with your knees bent and your feet flat on the floor, hip-width apart. Contract your abdominal muscles, pressing your lower back into the floor. Your pelvis should lift slightly off the floor. Hold for a few seconds, then relax into the starting position.

Do three to five repetitions.

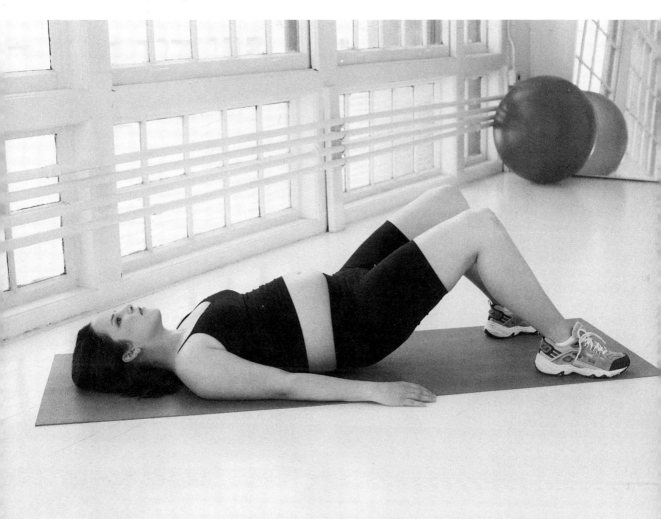

ONE-ARM DUMBBELL ROWS

Place your right leg on the center of a sturdy table or bench (about knee high). Your right hand should be braced on the bench. Your weight should be resting on your right knee and hand. Pick up a dumbbell in your left hand, palm facing toward you. Your left foot should be firmly on the ground. Keep your back flat. Lift the dumbbell, leading with your elbow, as high as you can toward your chest. Lower your arm back to the starting position. After one set, repeat with the opposite arm.

Do two sets of eight to ten repetitions.

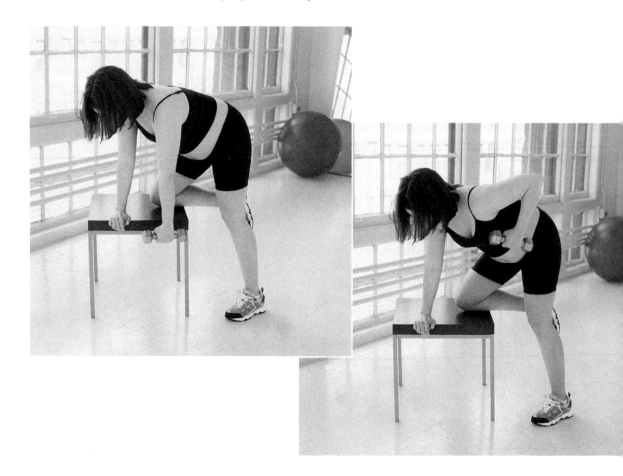

Tummy Toners

It is important to strengthen the muscles that you'll be using during labor. Before you can do that, you should be familiar with those muscles, especially the abdominals.

We have three sets of abdominals: the outer, inner, and middle layers. The rectus abdominus is the outermost layer. It contains two halves, called the recti. Due to the increase in size of the abdomen during pregnancy, it is quite common for the two halves to separate. This is called diastasis. You can check for it by lying on your back with your knees bent. (If you start to feel faint while on your back, roll onto your left side, then use pillows under your shoulders to prop yourself up.) Place your fingertips one to two inches below your belly button, fingers pointing toward your feet. Lifting your head as high as you can, see if you can feel a ridge protruding from the midline of your abdomen—that's a diastasis.

A one-to-two-finger-width gap is considered normal. A gap of more than two finger widths requires modifications to most of your abdominal exercises to keep the two halves of your abdomen from further separating.

When a diastasis of more than a two-finger-width separation exists, wrap a sheet (folded to about eight inches wide) around your waist and crisscross it in front of you to splint the abdomen when performing abdominal exercises. Hold on to the ends, and pull up and outward at a forty-five-degree angle as you contract your abdominal muscles, exhale, and raise your head and shoulders.

MODIFIED AB CRUNCH (IF YOU HAVE A DIASTASIS)

If you are past your first trimester, prop yourself up with pillows so your shoulders are higher than your belly. As described above, wrap a sheet around your waist and crisscross it in front. Don't knot it. Grasp and pull the ends up and outward at forty-five-degree angles as you contract your abdominal muscles, exhale, and raise your head. Do not lift shoulders.

Do one set of eight to twelve repetitions.

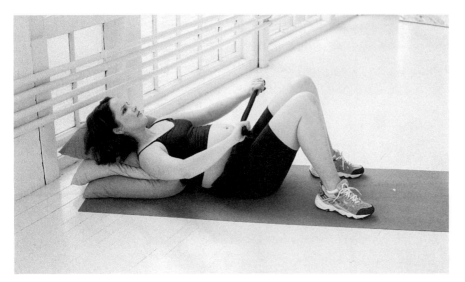

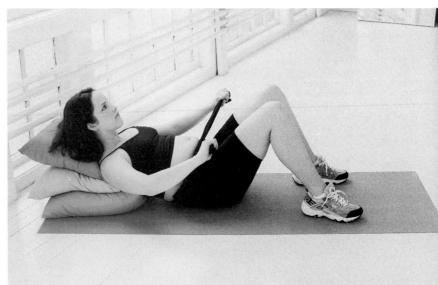

The following seven exercises are *not* recommended if you have a diastasis:

BRIDGE

Lie on a mat or carpeted surface, knees bent and feet flat on the floor. Place your arms by your sides, palms down. Tighten your abdominals and slowly lift your tailbone off the ground. As you lift higher, only your shoulder blades should be touching the floor. There should be a straight line running from your shoulders to your hips to your knees. Hold this position for ten seconds, then slowly lower to where your butt almost touches the ground. Repeat, slowly lifting your body. As pregnancy progresses, you may not be able to hold the position for ten seconds. If you feel any dizziness while on your back, discontinue the exercise.

Do two sets of eight to ten repetitions.

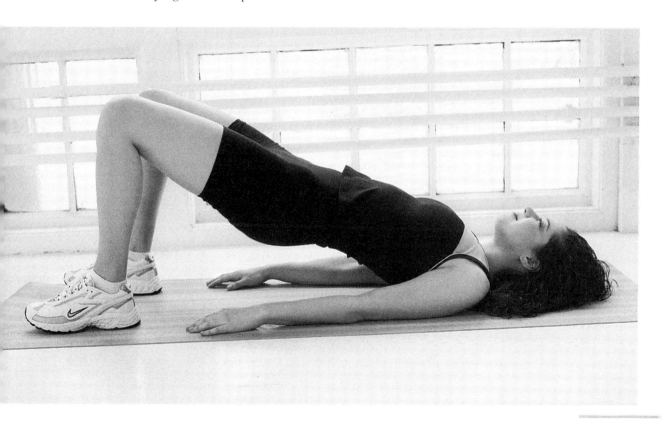

BALL ROLL

Kneeling, place your forearms and hands (clenched together) on a fitness ball. Your hips should be in line with your knees. Keeping your abdominals tight and back straight, roll forward about twelve inches, or until you feel a tightening in your abdominals. Pause, then slowly roll back to starting position. Make sure to maintain control when doing this exercise so the ball doesn't roll away.

Do two sets of eight to ten repetitions.

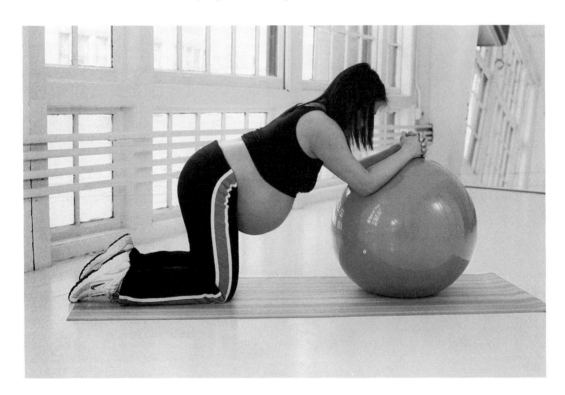

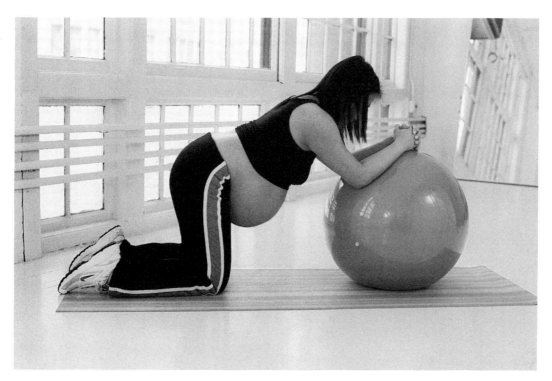

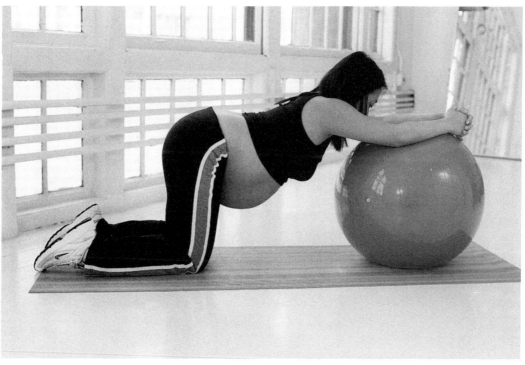

MODIFIED PLANK, FOREARMS AND KNEES— SECOND AND THIRD TRIMESTERS

Kneeling, place your forearms on the ground, shoulder-width apart. Inch your arms forward, keeping your back as straight as possible. Pull your abdominals in and tighten as you form a "plank."

Do two repetitions, holding each for ten to fifteen seconds.

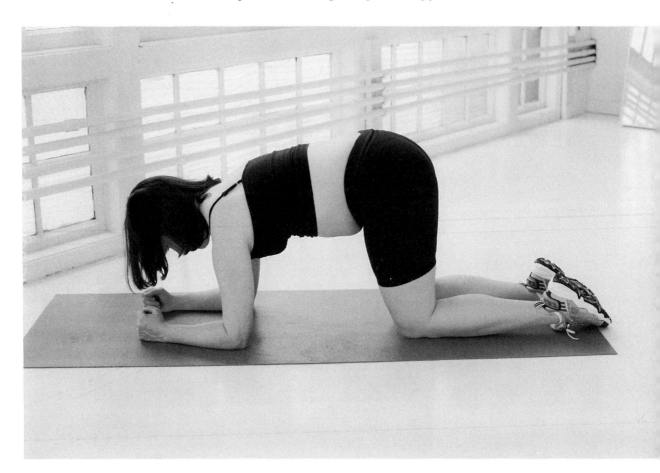

PLANK EXERCISES FOR FIRST AND EARLY SECOND TRIMESTERS

It is recommended that the following exercises be done only during the first and early second trimesters.

NONMODIFIED PLANK

Lie facedown on an exercise mat, with your elbows below your shoulders and your toes on the mat. Place one hand on top of the other so your forearms form a triangle. Tighten your abdominals and lift your entire body so it is now as straight as a plank and supported by your toes and elbows. Hold eight to fifteen seconds. Lower your body to the mat. Rest. Repeat.

If you have never done this exercise before, build your strength gradually. You may not be able to hold for eight seconds.

Avoid hunching your shoulders. Keep your shoulders open by pulling your shoulder blades together.

Do not allow your lower back to sag. Keep your abdominal muscles tight.

Keep breathing as you hold the position.

Do two repetitions, holding each for eight to fifteen seconds.

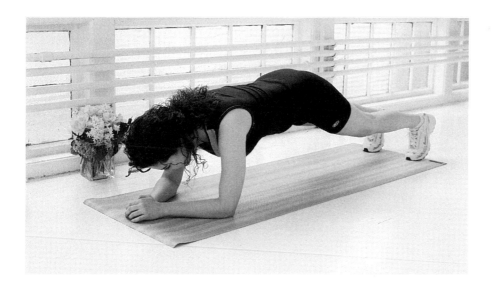

PLANK WITH BALL

From a kneeling position, pull a fitness ball in toward your quads, drape your torso over it, and put your hands on the floor in front of it. Tighten abs and walk hands forward until your hips are in front of the ball and your back is flat. Your feet will not be on the floor. This is the plank position. Continue to tighten your abs, letting the ball roll slightly under you toward your knees. Remember, the farther the ball is from your midsection, the more weight you will be supporting; the closer the ball is to your midsection, the more body weight the ball supports. Slowly return to neutral position by inching hands backward; toes will touch the floor.

Do two repetitions, trying to maintain the plank position for eight to ten seconds.

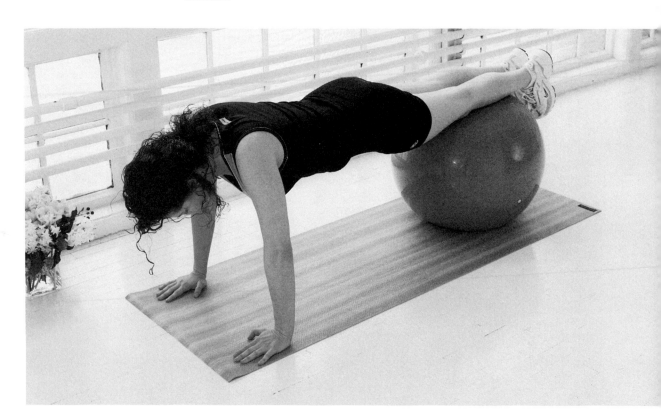

PLANK WITH BALL ROLL-IN

Begin from the plank position with the ball resting below your thighs, your abs tight and pulled in. Slowly let the ball roll down your thighs toward your lower legs, pulling your knees toward your chest. Hold for a second, then slowly roll the ball back to starting position.

Gradually build up your strength to complete eight to twelve repetitions.

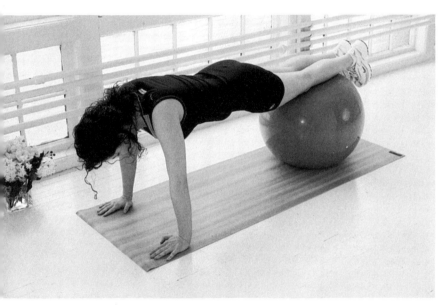

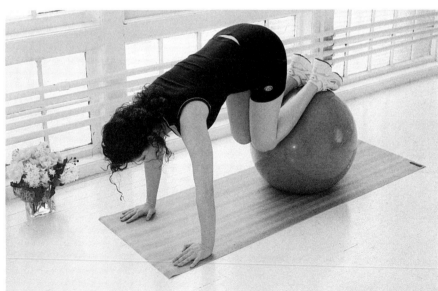

OBLIQUE SIDE RAISE

Lying on your right side, place your trunk on a fitness ball, allowing your trunk to slightly round the ball. Your right leg should be bent, left leg extended. Place your right hand at your temple and lightly rest your left arm on the front of the ball. Laterally flex and lift the left side of your trunk slowly, curling the rib cage toward the hip. Pause at the top of the movement, and then slowly return to starting position. Be sure to keep your head still and not roll forward or backward.

Do two sets of eight to ten repetitions.

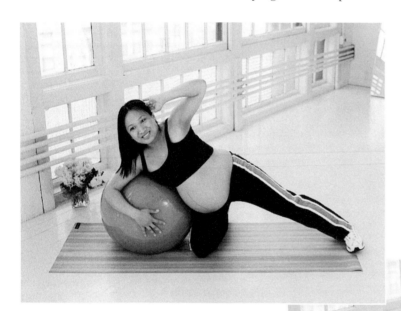

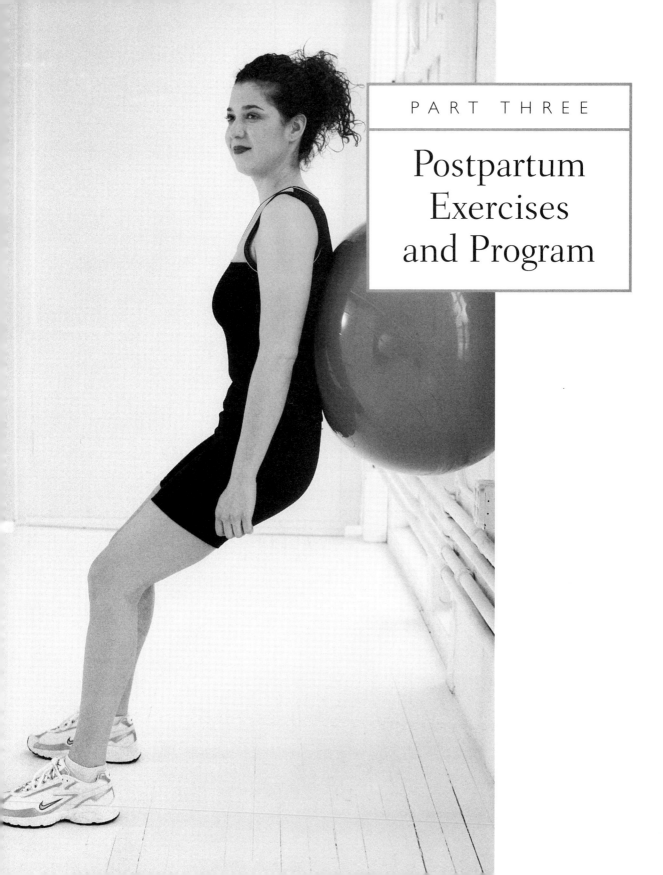

PART THREE

Postpartum
Exercises
and Program

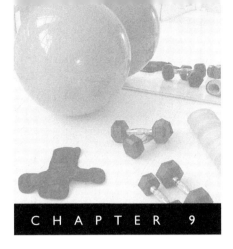

CHAPTER 9

Getting Your Body Back

POSTPARTUM EXERCISES: THE FIRST SIX WEEKS

Take It Slow

Congratulations—you just had a baby! So let's face it—getting back to your pre-baby exercise routine will take some time. Studies show that most women gain an average of twenty-five to thirty pounds during pregnancy. Most of this weight is lost a month after delivery. However, those last, stubborn ten pounds can be difficult to take off. But be consistent and patient. Strengthening of the abdominal and pelvic-floor muscles represents the foundation of a postpartum exercise program. During childbirth, the abdominal muscles are often stretched and the pelvic-floor muscles traumatized. Although the uterus will return to normal size within six weeks, specific strengthening exercises are required to restore the tone of the abdominal muscles. And though the abs may be the area you want to tone the most, the only way to shed remaining pregnancy pounds is by cardiovascular and aerobic exercise. Most obstetricians will tell you to wait until your six-week postpartum checkup. However, the American College of Obstetrics and Gynecology says it's OK to gradually resume an exercise routine based on your physical capabilities. Generally, if you exercised right up until delivery,

> ❧ *Before beginning any postpartum exercise routine, make sure to get the approval of your doctor.*

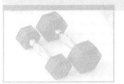

you can probably safely perform light exercises, such as modified sit-ups and stretching, right away. Walking is also an excellent way to get your body back. Short walks not only help with your cardiovascular endurance but also get you out of the house. Go slow, and don't push yourself.

Fitting exercise in during this hectic time may seem impossible. However, you should make it a priority if you are serious about getting back to your pre-pregnancy body.

Recent studies have indicated that moderate aerobic exercise performed four to five times a week postpartum has no adverse effect on lactation and significantly improves the cardiovascular fitness of mothers.

If you had a diastasis, make sure the gap in your stomach muscles has closed before progressing to abdominal exercises.

Your goal during the first six weeks after labor is to choose and perform a few exercises out of each group every other day. During the first two to three weeks, it's fine if you only do one exercise from each of the strength-training recommendations. You may do more, but only when you feel up to it. In the beginning, one set is recommended. Gradually build up to two sets when you feel stronger.

CESAREAN DELIVERY

Having a cesarean delivery can slow postpartum recovery. The desire to work out right away, especially if you were active during pregnancy, can be overwhelming. But I cannot stress enough the importance of refraining from strenuous exercise until your incisions have healed. Meet with your doctor and discuss what you can and cannot do during this important recovery time.

It is especially common to have the blues and mood changes following any delivery: your hormone levels have dropped significantly. Not being able to exercise can intensify those feelings. Be easy on yourself and don't hesitate to talk to your partner, friends, and medical professionals about your feelings.

Whether you had a difficult or easy labor, it is still possible to start some safe and simple exercises immediately after delivery. Keep a few things in mind, though. Your joints and ligaments are still stretched out and loose due to the relaxin in your body. Avoid sudden, quick movements the first few weeks after pregnancy, and allow your body to heal.

Most of all, give yourself time (and a break!) to return to your pre-pregnancy shape. Many women feel the effects of pregnancy up to a year after delivery. Just try to be patient and consistent, and let your body naturally recover and adjust.

WHERE TO START

If you are new to an exercise program or working out for the first time, concentrate more on short walks, light stretching, and abdominal tightening. Ease into a fitness routine. The goals described below are generally for new moms who safely performed some exercises during pregnancy.

Week 1

(The following information is recommended for women who had a regular and relatively easy labor. It is advised that women who had cesarean deliveries check with their doctor before starting any fitness program.)

Cardiovascular Goal

How do you feel? Are you able to get up and walk around with minimal discomfort? It the answer is yes, you are probably ready for a short walk around the block. You can even take your baby if you own a stroller. Start slow: about a five-to-seven-minute walk is best. Monitor how you feel. If you experience any shortness of breath or dizziness, stop immediately. If you feel good, try again during week 1. Two to three five-minute walks this first week is a great way to get back into the exercise world.

Kegel Exercises

Exercising in all three positions will make these muscles stronger. Even if you were doing Kegels while pregnant, you may not be able to hold the contraction as long postpartum. Start slow and gradually build up. Refer to pages 52–53 for effective Kegel instructions.

Abdominal Strengthening

It might seem unfair, but some women can get back into their pre-pregnancy shape in no time. But they're the exceptions; it may take a few months to get that flat tummy back. A lot depends on genes, how much weight you gained during pregnancy, and how active you were during pregnancy.

If you have a diastasis, before you do any abdominal work, make sure that you let your abdominals heal properly. Refer to page 87 for the correct technique in determining if you have a separation of the abdominal walls.

Abdominal Goals

ABDOMINAL TIGHTENING

Lying on your back, suck in your abdominals and hold for about three to five seconds. Release. During the first week, gradually work up to five seconds. It sounds easier than it really is.

Do eight to ten repetitions and two to three sets daily.

Lower-Back Strengthening

PELVIC TILTS

Lie on your back with your knees bent and your feet flat on the floor, hip-width apart. Contract your abdominal muscles, pressing your lower back into the floor. Your pelvis should lift slightly off the floor. Hold for five to ten seconds. Release.

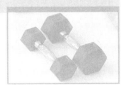

❯ Now that you've had your baby, you may want to watch the snacking, especially if you're not breast-feeding.

Week 2

Cardiovascular Goal

You should be feeling a bit stronger the second week after delivery. If you were able to take a couple of walks during the first week, you're doing great! During week 2, add a third walk to the week and try to stretch it to ten to twelve minutes. Don't push it, though; it's still very early and you don't want to jeopardize your recovery. I don't recommend any of the cardio options that I spoke about in Chapter 5. Stick to walking this week; you may able to mix it up during week 3.

Kegels

If you could only do one form of Kegel during week 1, you may feel strong enough this week to add a variation. Build on week 1, holding the Kegel ten to twelve seconds for each repetition.

Do three sets.

Abdominal Goal: Choose at Least Two

Continue with:

ABDOMINAL TIGHTENING

Add:

LEG SLIDES (RECOMMENDED IF YOU STILL DETECT A DIASTASIS AND IF YOU HAD A CESAREAN BIRTH)

Lying on your back, press your lower back against the floor by tightening your abdominal muscles. Keep your knees bent. Slide your left leg down so it's flat on the floor. Exhale, and bend back to starting position. Repeat with other leg. Make sure to keep your abs pressed into the floor throughout.

Do two sets of eight to ten repetitions.

BRIDGE (REFER TO PAGE 89):

Do one to two sets, six to eight repetitions.

BALL SITS

That's right, just sit on a fitness ball. The important thing to remember is to keep your back straight and abdominals tight. Your feet should be flat on the floor. This simple activity will improve your posture and help begin the process of tightening up the abs.

Lower-Back Goal: Choose at Least Two

Continue with:

PELVIC TILTS

Add:

HUGGIES

Lie flat on your back. Hug your knees to your chest and at the same time, bring your chin to your chest.
  Repeat twice, holding for ten seconds each.

Stretching

Stretching is a great way to relieve some of the tightness and soreness you may be experiencing after delivery. Your goal, every day, is to stretch all major muscle groups. Stretching is also recommended before and after each exercise session. Hold each stretch for ten to twenty seconds and be sure not to bounce. See Chapter 6 for effective stretches for the upper and lower body.

Pay extra attention to stretching muscles of the upper and lower back. And don't overstretch; your ligaments are still quite loose.

Week 3

Cardiovascular Goal

You should start to feel a lot of relief from the soreness of delivery during week 3. Again, don't push yourself too hard, but as you get stronger you may be able to do more vigorous exercise. Check your heart rate periodically during your program. If you're physically able, your walks can be longer, alternating a minute of jogging to every three minutes of walking. If you experience any abdominal pain, return to walking, picking up the pace. You can also resume biking (I'd stick with a stationary bike to avoid falls) and swimming. Keep these activities brief—ten to twelve minutes. You'll be amazed how you've lost your cardiovascular endurance, especially if you were quite active right up to delivery. Yoga is another great activity to incorporate back into your exercise plan. If you have no experience with yoga, there are plenty of entry-level classes taught by postpartum specialists. Many yoga studios offer babysitting services, with trained specialists. Take advantage of this opportunity to get out of the house.

It's especially crucial to begin each workout with a warm-up. Try a few minutes of walking in place or mini step-ups. Stretch, taking the time to target each muscle group.

Kegels

Continue with daily Kegel exercises, increasing the duration of each Kegel.

Strength Training

As you begin to add to your strengthening program, don't feel like you have to do *all* of the recommended goals and exercises. Pace yourself and gradually build up your endurance and strength. This is just a guideline to follow during your road to postpartum fitness.

Abdominal Goal: Choose at Least Two

Continue with:

LEG SLIDES

ABDOMINAL TIGHTENING

BALL SITS

BRIDGE

Add:

MODIFIED PLANK (REFER TO PAGE 92):

Do two sets, holding for eight to ten seconds.

Lower-Back Goals: Choose at Least Two

Continue with:

PELVIC TILTS

HUGGIES

Add:

CAT STRETCH (REFER TO PAGE 39)

Upper-Body Goals: Choose at Least One

**HAMMER CURLS ON BALL
(REFER TO PAGE 67)**

Do two sets of ten to twelve repetitions. Start off with very light weights.

TRICEPS EXTENSION (REFER TO PAGES 68–69)

Stretching

You should be able to hold each stretch for a longer duration and increase your range of motion. Target each muscle group.

Week 4

Cardiovascular Goal

You're doing great! Just keep monitoring how you feel. Try walking for twenty to thirty minutes at a brisk pace three times a week. If you're a runner, add some slow jogging into your walks, and continue with the pattern of walking/jogging. Increase the jogging-to-walking ratio to 1.5 to 2 minutes of jogging to 2 minutes of walking. Some women may find this very easy, especially if their pregnancy was not complicated. On the other hand, running for two minutes still may be extremely difficult. If you can't have a conversation while jogging, you're pushing yourself too much. Stick to more walking, increasing the pace.

Kegels

Daily Kegels will further strengthen your pelvic-floor muscles. If you are consistent, you should see a difference in your ability to control bladder leaks, in the healing of the perineum, and in tightening of the vagina, which will be stretched from birth.

Do fifteen to twenty times in a row, three to five times a day.

Abdominal Goal: Choose at Least Three

Continue with:

LEG SLIDES

ABDOMINAL TIGHTENING

BALL SITS

BRIDGE

MODIFIED PLANK

Add:

CURL-UPS

Lying on your back on an exercise mat or carpeted surface, bend your knees and place your feet flat on the floor. Contract your abs, lifting your head, neck, and shoulder blades off the floor. Trying not to jerk your body, raise it to the count of three. Lower to the count of three.

Do two sets of ten to twelve repetitions.

Lower-Back/Back Goal: Choose at Least Two, Switching Exercises Every Other Day

Continue with:

PELVIC TILTS

HUGGIES

CAT STRETCHES

Add:

SUPER MOMS

Lying facedown on a mat or carpet, extend your legs, toes pointed. Extend your arms over your head. Look forward, keeping your head steady, your chin off the ground.

Slowly raise your left arm and right leg at the same time until they are a few inches off the ground. Slowly lower to starting position. Repeat with your right arm and left leg.

Lower-Body/Leg Goal: Choose at Least Two, Switching Exercises Every Other Day

You should be feeling strong enough at this time to incorporate strength training for your arms and legs. To start, use three-to-five-pound dumbbells. To increase difficulty, add repetitions and/or an additional set.

Add:

DUMBBELL SQUATS (REFER TO PAGE 74)

Do one set of ten to twelve repetitions.

CALF RAISES OFF STEP (REFER TO PAGE 80)

Start off with your own body weight. If you find this easy, add light weight, three-to-five-pound dumbbells.

Do one set of ten to twelve repetitions.

ADDUCTOR SQUEEZE WITH PILLOW (REFER TO PAGE 82)

Do two sets of eight to ten repetitions.

Upper-Body Goal: Choose at Least Three, Switching Exercises Every Other Day

Continue with:

HAMMER CURLS ON BALL

TRICEPS EXTENSIONS

Add:

MODIFIED PUSH-UPS (REFER TO PAGE 58)

Start slow and easy. One set is fine to start. Make sure you have a good base of support, keeping your knees and hands shoulder-width apart.

ALTERNATING ARM RAISES (REFER TO PAGE 62)

Do one to two sets with three-to-five-pound weights.

Stretching

Continue with daily stretching.

Weeks 5 through 6 and beyond

Cardiovascular Goal

At the six-week mark, you should be getting back into the swing of things. Again, all pregnancies are different, and you may still be very uncomfortable and tired. Just because it's been six weeks doesn't mean you should ignore those feelings and dive into an exercise program. Monitoring your perceived rate of exertion is important. You can start to increase the time and intensity of cardiovascular activities, elevating your heart rate, trying to get near your target-heart-rate zone. However, be conscious of your energy levels. A lot of women don't even think about exercising until the six-week point. Six weeks usually marks the time when you visit your doctor and check in on how you're feeling. Keep your doctor abreast of your current fitness program and what you intend to do over the course of the next few weeks and months. Discuss any personal fitness goals you may have, so your doctor can monitor you effectively. Experienced runners may find that they're able to run continuously for ten to twelve minutes without stopping to walk. Swimmers may be able to add a few more laps to their workout. If you're up to getting the bike out of the garage, now is a good time to get out of the house and ride around the neighborhood. Stay with smooth terrains. Investigate some of the postnatal fitness classes that focus on cardiovascular activities and stretching.

As far as strength training is concerned, feel free to try any of the exercises described in Chapter 7. If any one feels uncomfortable or you just don't feel strong enough, take your time and wait a couple more weeks. With time and a stronger body, you'll be able to safely add all of the exercises into your weekly workouts. If the weight recommendations are too light or too heavy, adjust them to your comfort level and ability. If you are doing some of the strength-training exercises for the first time, start with light weights, or use your own body weight in the beginning. Again, these are general recommendations. Finally, as you start to get back to your normal fitness routine, develop a program that works for you. You may not be able to do some of your regular exercises for a few more weeks or even months. Be patient, don't overexert yourself, and most of all, stay consistent. Results take time, especially for new moms.

Kegels

Those Kegel exercise should be paying off. Keep up with the daily strengthening techniques.

Abdominal Goals: Choose at Least Four, Switching Exercises Every Other Day

Continue with:

LEG SLIDES

ABDOMINAL TIGHTENING

BALL SITS

BRIDGE

MODIFIED PLANK

CURL-UPS

Add:

BALL ROLL (REFER TO PAGE 90)

Do one to two sets of eight to ten repetitions.

OBLIQUE SIDE RAISES

Do one to two sets of eight to ten repetitions.

PLANK

As you get stronger, you'll be able to hold the plank position for longer periods of time.

Lower-Back/Upper-Back Goals: Choose Two, Switching Exercises Every Other Day

Continue with:

PELVIC TILTS

HUGGIES

CAT STRETCH

Add:

ONE-ARM DUMBBELL ROWS (REFER TO PAGE 86)

Start with five-pound dumbbells, until you feel stronger.
   Do two sets of eight to ten repetitions.

*Legs/Lower-Body Goals: Choose at Least Three,
Switching Exercises Every Other Day*

Continue with:

DUMBBELL SQUATS

CALF RAISES OFF STEP

ADDUCTOR SQUEEZE WITH PILLOW

Add:

BUTT LIFTS

STEP-UPS WITH BENCH

ABDUCTOR LEG LIFT

KNEELING LEG LIFT

WALL SITS WITH BALL

*Arms/Upper-Body Goals: Choose at Least Four,
Switching Exercises Every Other Day*

Continue with:

HAMMER CURLS ON BALL

TRICEPS EXTENSIONS

MODIFIED PUSH-UPS

ALTERNATING ARM RAISES

Add:

ALTERNATING BICEPS CURLS (PAGE 66)

Do two sets of ten to twelve repetitions using five-to-eight-pound weights.

UPWARD ROWS (REFER TO PAGE 63)

Do one to two sets of eight to ten repetitions using five-to-eight-pound weights.

OVERHEAD PRESS ON BALL (REFER TO PAGE 61)

Do one to two sets of eight to ten repetitions using five-to-eight-pound weights.

TRICEPS DIPS (REFER TO PAGE 70)

Do one set of eight to ten repetitions.

CHEST PRESS WITH BALL, OR FLAT SURFACE (REFER TO PAGE 60)

If you find that doing this exercise on a fitness ball places too much strain on you, use a flat bench or a mat on the floor in place of the ball.

Do one set of eight to ten repetitions, using an eight-to-ten-pound weight.

Activities With Your Baby

CRUNCHES FOR TOTS

Lie on your back, bend your knees to your chest, and place your baby right below your knees. Lift your head and shoulders enough to clear the floor; try not to use your neck/head to help you lift. You'll feel this burn those abdominal muscles, plus your baby will love the rocking motion.

BABY BENCH PRESS

Lying on a carpeted floor (or exercise mat), hold your baby in both hands and extend your arms straight up. Try not to lock your arms, then slowly lower to starting position. This exercise is great for strengthening the chest muscles.

LULLABY LUNGES

Placing your baby in a stroller, grab the handle firmly with your left hand, with the stroller to your left. Your feet should be shoulder-width apart and your abdominals tight. With your right foot, take a step forward. Your left leg should be almost straight. Slowly lower your body by bending your right leg. Be sure to keep the right knee over the right toes when lowering. Just before your left knee touches the ground, slowly push up. Then take a step forward with your left foot, repeating the same motion. At the same time you should be gently pushing the stroller forward.

Targets quadriceps, butt, hamstrings.

TODDLER TWISTS

Sitting on an exercise mat or carpeted floor, cross your legs and hold your baby with both hands. Extend your arms out and gently twist your body to your right, bringing both your head and baby to your right side. Pause, then twist to your left side.

Targets abdominal muscles, obliques.

Cardiovascular Activities

When your baby is around six months of age and has better head control and strength, take him/her out for a jog or cycle in a jog stroller or bike trailer.

The important thing to remember during all of this is to be gentle on yourself and listen to your doctor. Keep yourself strong and healthy by eating right. Don't be afraid to ask for help from your partner, family, and friends to catch up on your sleep. Stay well hydrated, and don't give up. You will lose the baby weight, but it will take some time and commitment. Good luck, and congratulations . . . you're now a Buff Mom!

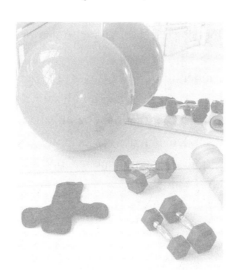

Acknowledgments

No matter what accomplishments you achieve, someone always helps you. That holds true for the making of this book. I am deeply grateful to so many wonderful people who have given me their support throughout this project. Thank you to the extremely talented people at Random House, especially Bruce Tracy, my editor Danielle Durkin, and publicist Kate Blum. A special thank-you to Ivan Held, Mary Bahr, and Kimberly Burns, for ultimately making this book a reality.

I want to express my appreciation to the many contributors to the book, especially the model Julie Stark, model moms Jean Cabacungan-Jarvis and Sara Schneider, and cover mom Alison Rich. Thank you to photographer Joan Lauren for your vision and beautiful photography, Jenn Kennedy for your exceptional talent and flattering author photograph, Jack Myers and Dan Rembert for your brilliant eye and creativity in designing the cover, and Carol Myers at Divine Studio in New York for your breathtaking studio space. Thank you to Lisa Hufcut, Libby Clark, and New York Sports Clubs. Special thanks goes to my astute lawyer, Karen Shatzkin.

I am truly grateful for the amazing friendships of both colleagues and friends. Thank you to the many supportive people at the Riverdale Country School, especially Beth Norman, Kathy Schoonmaker, Lynn Sorenson, Tonia Maschi, David Hooks, and Kent Kildahl. I also express my deep gratitude to my amazing friends Suzanne Borda, Anita Cochran, Lauren Van Kirk, and Deb Larkin; special agents Gretchen Koss, Polly Defrank, and Bonnie Eldon; Sandra DeOvando and Pamela Guyer. Your endless friendship and support are invaluable. And, finally, thank you to Kate Frucher for sharing your love, kindness, and smile. It is truly a gift.

INDEX

A

abdomen/abdominal muscles
  and body changes during pregnancy, 10
  as part of core muscle group, 49
  and postpartum exercises, 99, 101, 102, 103–4, 106, 108, 112–13
  sets of, 87
  strengthening of, 54–56, 102
  stretching of, 7
  tightening of, 101, 102, 103, 106, 108, 112
  tips about, 56
  toning of, 54–56, 87–96
  See also diastasis
abductor leg lift, 83, 114
adductor squeeze with pillow, 82, 110, 114
adrenaline, 6
aerobic activities, 18, 25, 26, 99, 100. *See also* cardiovascular activities
alternating arm raises, 62, 110, 115
alternating biceps curls, 66, 115
alternating quadriceps lunges, 77
American College of Obstetrics and Gynecology (ACOG), 8, 12, 20, 99
ankle weights, 50, 79, 81, 83
arms/arm muscles
  alternating raising of, 62, 110, 115
  and postpartum exercises, 109, 110, 114–15
  strengthening of, 109

stretching of, 54
See also shoulder exercises

B

baby
  activities with, 116–17
  transporting, 7
baby bench press, 116
back
  aches in, 15
  exercises for upper, 105, 113
  lying on, 12, 13, 27, 30, 35, 54, 55, 89
  must-do exercises for, 84–86
  stretches, 54
  and weight training, 54
  See also lower back
balance, 26, 49, 68, 77, 83
ball, fitness
  ball roll with, 90–91, 112
  butt lifts with, 78
  chest press with, 60, 115
  concentration curl on, 65
  and creating home gym, 49
  and exercise tips, 56
  hammer curls on, 67, 107, 110, 114
  leg curl with, 72–73
  overhead press with, 61, 115
  plank exercises with, 94, 95
  push-ups with, 59

ball, fitness (*cont'd*):
    sitting on, 104, 106, 108, 112
    triceps extension on, 68, 69
    wall sits with, 76, 114
bench/step
    and baby bench press, 116
    calf raises off, 80, 110, 114
    and creating home gym, 50
    postpartum exercises with, 114, 115, 116
    step-ups with, 75, 114
    and strengthening and toning lower body,
        80
biceps curls, alternating, 66, 115
biking, 26, 27, 105, 111
bleeding, abnormal, 9
blood pressure, 8
body changes, 9–11
Borg's Scale of Perceived Exertion, 20, 21
Braxton Hicks contractions, 14, 54–55
breasts, 10
breathing
    appropriate, 57
    and body changes during pregnancy, 9
    during cardiovascular exercises, 57, 101
    guidelines about, 17
    and lying on back, 12
    and strength training, 57
    in third trimester, 15
    and weights, 55
bridge, 89, 104, 106, 108, 112
butt lifts, 78, 114

C

calf, exercises for, 24, 32, 80, 110, 114
cardiovascular activities
    and activities with baby, 117
    breathing during, 57, 101
    as element in fitness routine, 18
    and heart rate, 21
    and postpartum exercises, 23, 99, 100, 101,
        103, 105, 107, 111–12, 117
    safe, 23–26
    and stretching, 27
    variation in, 18
cat stretches, 39, 106, 109, 113
cesarean delivery, 100–101, 103
checklist, 56
chest/shoulder exercises, 41, 43, 54, 60, 115

circulation, 6
clothing, workout, 18, 21, 56
concentration curl on ball, 65
concentric phase, 55
constipation, 10, 14
contractions, 14, 25, 54–55
cool downs, 25, 54, 56
core muscle group, 49
core strength, 26, 49
crunches for tots, 116
curl-ups, 108, 112

D

deltoids/shoulders stretches, 43
diabetes, 8, 11, 14
diastasis, 57, 87, 88, 89, 100, 102, 103
diet, 12, 14, 18
dizziness
    from lying on back, 12, 13, 27, 30, 35,
        89
    and postpartum exercises, 101
    and stretching and running, 25
doctors, discussions with, 8, 17, 56, 99, 100,
        101, 111
dumbbells
    and back exercises, 86
    and creating home gym, 48
    with lower body exercises, 74, 75, 76,
        77
    one-arm dumbbell rows, 86, 113
    postpartum exercises with, 109, 110, 113,
        114
    squats with, 74, 109, 114
    with upper body exercises, 60–69, 71

E

eccentric phase, 55
emotions, 5–6, 13
energy, 6, 12–13, 14, 25, 111
estrogen, 10
exercise mats, 50
exercise program
    avoidance of, 8
    benefits of, 5–7, 15
    and body changes, 9–11
    guidelines for, 8–9, 17–18
    tips for, 56
    warning signs during, 9

postpartum exercises (*cont'd*):
  aerobic exercise as, 100
  for arms, 109, 110, 114–15
  with bench/step, 114, 115, 116
  and benefits of exercise, 7
  cardiovascular, 23, 99, 100, 101, 103, 105,
      107, 111–12, 117
  and cesarean delivery, 100–101
  for first six weeks, 99–115
  for legs, 103, 106, 108, 109, 112, 114
  and lower back, 102, 104, 105, 106, 109,
      113
  and lower body, 109–10, 114
  and strength training, 99, 102, 105–6, 109,
      111–12
  and stretches, 100, 101, 104–5, 107,
      111
  for upper back, 105
  for upper body, 107, 110, 114–15
  walking for, 100, 101, 105, 107
  and weight loss, 6
  with weights/dumbbells, 109, 110, 111–12,
      113, 114, 115
prayer stretch, 38
progesterone, 10
push-ups, 58, 59, 110, 114

Q
quadriceps exercises, 24, 28, 29, 77

R
relaxin, 10, 15, 18, 24, 101
repetition, 54, 55
running, 23–25, 105, 107, 111

S
second trimester, 13–14, 24–25, 70, 92,
    93–96
self-image, 6
serotonin, 5–6
sets, 55
shoulder exercises, 41, 43, 54, 60,
    115
side leg lift, 81
sit-ups, 56, 100
sitting glutes stretches, 36
sleep, 6, 15
sneakers, 24

spine, exercises for, 37, 49
squats, 55, 56, 74, 109, 114
step aerobics, 25
step-ups, 55, 75, 114
stomach. *See* abdomen/abdominal
    muscles
strength training
  abdominal, 54, 102
  for arms, 109
  beginning, 47–48
  and body changes during pregnancy,
      11
  breathing during, 57
  creating home gym for, 48–50
  as element in fitness routine, 18
  for legs, 109
  for lower back, 49, 102
  for lower body, 72–83
  and postpartum exercises, 99, 102, 105–6,
      109, 111–12
  for upper body, 57–71
  and warm ups and cool downs, 54
  and weights, 54
  and what to expect during pregnancy,
      15
  See also weights
stretches
  and aerobics, 25
  arm/shoulder, 54
  back, 54
  calf, 24, 32
  checklist concerning, 56
  chest, 54
  as element in fitness routine, 18
  guidelines about, 18
  hamstring, 24, 30, 31
  leg/thigh, 33, 54
  lower back, 15, 24, 37–39, 105
  lower body, 28–36
  overview about, 27
  and postpartum exercises, 100, 101, 104–5,
      107, 111
  quadriceps, 24, 28
  and running, 24–25
  and swimming, 25
  for upper back, 105
  for upper body, 40–43
  and warm ups and cool downs, 27, 54

and what to expect in first trimester, 13

super moms, 109

supine hypotensive syndrome, 12

swimming, 25, 105, 111

T

target heart rate (THR), 20–23, 111

thigh stretches, 33

third trimester, 15–16, 24–25, 92

tips, exercise program, 56

toddler twists, 117

toning

lower body, 72–83

upper body, 57–71

See also weights

triceps exercises, 41, 42, 68, 69, 70, 71, 107, 110, 114, 115

tummy toners, 87–96

U

upper back exercises, 105, 113

upper body

postpartum exercises for, 107, 110, 114–15

strengthening and toning of, 57–71

stretches for, 40–43

upward rows, 63, 115

urination, 10

uterus, 9, 10, 13, 14, 15

V

vitamins, 13

W

walking/power walking, 13, 23, 24, 27, 100, 101, 103, 105, 107

wall sits with ball, 76, 114

warm ups, 25, 27, 54, 56, 105

warning signs, 9

water/fluids

and body temperature, 21–22

and exercise, 57

guidelines about, 18

and stretching and running, 25

and what to expect during pregnancy, 12, 13, 14

weight, and body changes during pregnancy, 10

weights

ankle, 50, 79, 81, 83

and lying on back, 54

overview about, 54–56

postpartum exercises with, 110, 111–12, 115

and strengthening and toning upper body, 79, 81, 83

See also dumbbells

Y

Yoga, 105

ABOUT THE AUTHOR

SUE FLEMING earned her B.S. and M.S. in physical education and has been a certified personal trainer for the past ten years. The author of *Buff Brides* (now a series on the Discovery Health Channel) and *Buff Moms,* she is currently the director of physical education at Riverdale Country School in Riverdale, New York, and continues to work with private clients. She lives in Manhattan. Sue Fleming can be reached at www.buffbrides.com.

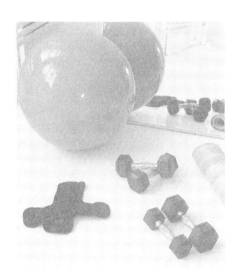